THE NEW FERTILITY AND CONCEPTION

The Essential Guide for Childless Couples

Everyone has heard myths and half-truths about producing a pregnancy. Sometimes the apparent problems that a couple experience are based on these erroneous assumptions and nothing more. This comprehensive guide explains the process of normal human reproduction, where it may go wrong, and what can be done about it. Dr. John J. Stangel, a distinguished professional, furnishes the essential information for every couple seeking alternatives to childlessness.

JOHN J. STANGEL, M.D., is a physician whose entire professional life has been directed toward treating and solving problems of reproduction. He is the Medical Director of IVF America—Westchester at United Hospital, Port Chester, New York, and a Clinical Associate Professor in the Department of Obstetrics and Gynecology at New York Medical College. He also maintains a clinical practice in Rye, New York, devoted entirely to infertility and other reproductive problems. Dr. Stangel is ~~~~~~~~~ ~~~~~~ aged in research and publication

D1261964

THE NEW FERTILITY AND CONCEPTION

The Essential Guide
for Childless Couples

BY
JOHN J. STANGEL, M.D.

With a Foreword by

Martin L. Stone, M.D.
Past President of the
American College
of Obstetricians and Gynecologists

Library of Congress Cataloging-in-Publication Data

Stangel, John J., 1941–
    The new fertility and conception : the essential guide for childless
couples / by John J. Stangel : with a foreword by Martin
L. Stone.—Rev. and updated ed.
    p. cm.
Rev. ed. of: Fertility and conception. 1979.
ISBN 0-452-26005-1
  1. Infertility. 2. Conception. 3. Human reproduction.
4. Fertility, Human. I. Stangel, John J., 1941– Fertility and
conception. II. Title.
RC889.S63 1988
616.6'92—dc19   87-32060
                                                                CIP

First Printing, Revised and Updated Edition, June, 1988

1 2 3 4 5 6 7

PRINTED IN THE UNITED STATES OF AMERICA

To Lois, my wife and my closest friend

To my patients, who have shared their problems and feelings with me and have taught me a great deal—more than any textbook—and who have allowed me the privilege of treating them

To my mother, Regina, and my father, Abraham, who gave me life, love, and support and who taught me who I am

and

To my sons, Justin and Eric, who have given me the joy, wonder, and excitement of seeing the world through their eyes

Acknowledgments

IT WOULD be impossible to list and thank all the people whose thoughts and work have influenced this book. To all who have contributed through their writing, research, or personal communication, I wish to express my appreciation. There are a few without whose specific assistance this volume would not be a reality. In this connection I wish to thank Richard Resnick, M.D., Walter L. Freedman, M.D., J. Victor Reyniak, M.D., Harry Settles, Ph.D., Carlton Eddy, Ph.D., Sidney Shulman, Ph.D., and Linsey Levine. For their help in the preparation of the second edition of this book I wish to thank Patricia Mazzola, Ronald Batt, M.D., Richard Bronson, M.D., James Daniell, M.D., Michael Wenof, M.D., Carl Wood, M.D., Alan Trounson, Ph.D., and their coinvestigators at Monash University; and Bob Moses, Floyd Willison, Vicki Baldwin, Kathryn Honea, M.D., Sheldon Lippert, M.D., Anthony Lioacono, M.D., Robert Madison, M.D., Joel Novendstern, M.D., Albert Parker, M.D., Ronald Reiss, M.D., Pedro Rojas, M.D., and Donna Howlett, all of IVF America. I want to thank Angela Miller, David Gibbons, and Alexia Dorszynski, without whose efforts this second edition would not have been published. I want to express my appreciation to Jeanne Lolya and Lois Stangel for preparing the manuscript. Finally, I wish to thank my wife, Lois, for her constant patience, encouragement, and support.

Contents

Preface

THIS PREFACE is our expression of thanks to Dr. John Stangel and, we hope, a beacon of encouragement for all who read this book.

Our encounter with infertility began five years ago. It was to become a process of experiences which would take us through most of the spectrum of human emotion. At first, there was frustration and a nagging fear that something was wrong, as we attempted, unsuccessfully, to conceive on our own. When it became time, a year later, for a fertility workup, there was already anger and desperation. The waiting involved in every step was excruciating—waiting for a period, waiting for a doctor's appointment, waiting for the right time of the month for a test, and waiting for a result, with fear and hope strangely mixed together. Our fear of finding something really wrong combined with our hope that something treatable would be found.

The first problem discovered was treatable with medication and we grew encouraged. We were to learn that our monthly routine would require adjustments of medication and analysis of the response. Though there was careful medical adjustment and continued patience on our part, each onset of menstruation brought disappointment and despair. However, each also signaled a beginning, a new chance. Hope replaced gloom, usually within a day or two.

Pressure built and stress grew: procedures and new treatments had to fit between busy work schedules; our marriage, once a blend of love, careers, and home, was now solely an obsession. It seemed, too, that few friends could understand the depth of our obsession, and we began to feel apart and isolated.

Our efforts continued for several more years with both male and female problems. In our case, as soon as the female factors seemed appropriately treated, treatment of the male factor began. We watched, with mixed emotions, as many other couples achieved eventual success following their treatments. Despite the frustrations and, at times, deep discouragement, we trudged on. Why? Part of the reason was surely human nature, and part was intellectual. We knew from experience that each effort we made brought refinements and improvements in our doctor's treatment strategy. We also knew that the advances in the field were growing at an astounding rate, and that our doctor was out on the frontline of this knowledge. There were times that our treatment was changed on a monthly basis because of new discoveries. There was hope for us because we knew that we were on the cutting edge of the latest medical advances. We never abandoned the image of our baby, and we never wavered in our faith and trust of our doctor.

After the fourth year of our quest, Dr. Stangel informed us that he was to become the medical director of a new in vitro fertilization program and that we could be candidates. Once again, new hope was given to us.

We began our fifth year of hope by attempting an IVF cycle. Although faced with additional unexpected problems, we completed the cycle with the transfer of three embryos. Merely to get eggs, and to know that they had been fertilized and developed into embryos, was uplifting and exhilarating. The more we learned, the more we could hope. We waited the required two weeks, braced for the results . . . and were told it had not worked.

We were determined to try again.

> Gail and Leonard Maisel
> Westchester, N.Y.
> January 1987

Gail Maisel delivered a healthy baby in July of 1987.

Foreword

THIS VERY timely book deals with infertility, its causes, diagnosis, and treatment. It is up to date and current in covering the field at a time when new directions are being charted daily.

The author, who is both knowledgeable and experienced, has produced a readable text for the nonprofessional. With skill he blends an unusual sensitivity and understanding of his patients and their needs with the scientific advances occurring so rapidly.

The format is innovative and interesting, the diagrams clear and most helpful. The result is an unusually complete and extensive text that is still easy to follow and understand. Dr. Stangel covers not only the mechanistic approaches used to investigate and treat the infertile couple but also the role of life-style factors such as stress and exercise. The latest research developments are thoroughly covered, and their implications discussed.

This excellent book will be of real value to the couple who has an infertility problem and to their physician, since the couple's understanding of the problem will make the doctor's efforts to help more productive. Even those who have no reproductive problems will find this an informative and useful text.

MARTIN L. STONE. M.D.,
Professor and Chairman,
Department of Obstetrics and Gynecology,
State University of New York at Stony Brook, and
President of the American College of
Obstetricians and Gynecologists (1979)

Introduction

I SAT behind my desk on a bright spring afternoon. A woman in her late twenties sat across from me, shifted in her seat and continued talking. "I am tired of trying for something that other people take for granted. My friends are all getting pregnant and I'm not. Many of the women on my street are pregnant for the third and fourth time because they have nothing better to do, and I can't do it even once. I feel resentful when I walk down the street and see other women pushing baby carriages. Jeff and I have tried for so long that I just can't stand it any longer. Sex used to be one of the most enjoyable things in our lives but now it has become a mechanical chore. When the time for my period approaches I wait with anticipation and dread. We are good people. Our home is full of love. I feel we would make wonderful parents, but it just doesn't seem to happen."

I hear this call for help almost daily. The person speaking and the words change a bit, but each time the feelings are just as desperate. These are the feelings of a couple trying unsuccessfully to have a child. Though not always discussed openly and freely, infertility is more common than one might imagine. Our country is filled with people who are concerned with overpopulation and who spend money preventing or terminating unwanted pregnancies. For them, having children is so easy that they need scarcely think about it. Few realize that 15 percent of couples trying to have a child are unable to do so, and that this percentage may

1

rise. When stories are told at social gatherings we may hear about couples who have had immediate success achieving pregnancy. People tend not to speak of what they feel to be their failures. It is very likely that in any group of ten couples of reproductive age at least one person in the room has a reproductive problem or personally knows someone with such a difficulty.

One out of six married couples seeks the aid of a physician because of infertility. Following infertility evaluation, the cause of the problem can be determined in about 93 percent of cases. Nearly 80 percent of treated couples conceive, and this percentage is increasing.

Unlike many other medical problems, infertility is a problem of couples, not individuals. Both members are affected even though only one member may have a physical problem. As a result, infertility tests the very fiber of intimate human relationships.

We have been taught myths and half-truths about producing a pregnancy and occasionally the apparent problems that a couple might experience are based on these errors and nothing more. The purpose of this book is to dispel some of these myths, to explain the process of normal human reproduction, where it may go wrong and what can be done about it.

Great strides have been made in the diagnosis and treatment of infertility in the last few years and this is just the beginning. There is more hope today than ever before.

We are about to start on the long road of investigation and treatment which we hope, will have at its end the birth of a normal, healthy baby. It is frequently a difficult trip because it is drawn out over several weeks or months and different tests must be timed at various times of the woman's menstrual cycle. Sometimes the test results, instead of answering questions, pose more questions and require further studies. After we reach a diagnosis and begin treatment, more time must pass to see if treatment is successful. Since ovulation usually occurs only once a month, many months may pass before we see results. This often means that the time necessary to achieve a pregnancy while under treatment for infertility becomes difficult to bear. There are many things couples should know to help sustain them through the evaluation and treatment period. But it is a rare patient who manages to ask all his or her questions, or who can absorb all the information offered by the physician. Often this is results of the stress of being in a doctor's office.

This book is an attempt to offer what I feel is the essential information infertile couples need to deal with their problems. By understanding why and how tests are done and how these tests really feel, you can tolerate them more easily. By understanding why tests are scheduled when they are in relation to your menstrual cycle, the delays in completing the investigation are less frustrating. By learning how different modes of treatment work, the fact that you may not achieve pregnancy immediately is no longer surprising and therefore may be less depressing. By possessing all the information, we can deal with the road to pregnancy with greater ease.

This book is written in "layers" so that it is possible to get a brief discussion of a topic by reading the opening paragraphs, or to get a more extensive explanation of a topic by reading further. Basic ideas and important concepts are repeated from chapter to chapter for emphasis and to make understanding easier, and to reduce the necessity of turning back and forth from chapter to chapter. Illustrations and charts are used extensively to expand and support the discussions.

In addition, you will find a large glossary of terms at the back of the book. Use it when you do not understand a term that I or any other practitioner uses.

Let us now take the first step in our journey.

CHAPTER 1
A Matter of Terms

BEFORE DISCUSSING anything in detail, it is always important to understand the vocabulary to be used. Infertility is certainly no exception. The purpose of this chapter is to lay the groundwork for the discussions to follow in the next several chapters by presenting the most important terms, defining and then discussing them. Then, I will present male and female anatomy and briefly review their relevance to infertility.

DEFINITIONS

Infertility is the inability of a heterosexual couple to produce a pregnancy after one year of regular intercourse. For a short sentence this definition has a fair number of qualifications in it. It does not simply say that infertility is the inability of two people to have children. It sets a limit on the amount of time that a couple must try and implies a certain frequency of sexual intercourse. Approximately 80 percent of sexually active couples of reproductive age will conceive within one year. If an infertility evaluation is begun before a year has passed, many couples with no reproductive problem will be studied unnecessarily. In order to achieve pregnancy a certain number of tries must be made within one year so that there is enough chance for fertilization to occur. Making love every other month for a year would not allow sufficient sexual exposure and would be an inadequate trial of a couple's fertility. Most experts say that a couple should have intercourse approximately every other day around the time of ovulation or every other day throughout the cycle, every month for twelve months without achieving pregnancy before they consider an infertility evaluation.

Another use of the word "infertility" refers to the inability of the woman to carry a pregnancy through to the delivery of a live birth. A pregnancy ending in the loss of a fetus before it is able to survive on its own is referred to as a *miscarriage* or an *abortion*. Note that the medical use of the word "abortion" simply means the loss of a pregnancy before it can survive. It does not imply that the pregnancy was ended by medication or surgical manipulation.

Abortions may be described as *spontaneous*, that is, occurring without any manipulation or the administration of medication; or *induced*, implying that something has been done to cause the loss of the pregnancy. The medical definition of *habitual abortion* is spontaneous loss of three consecutive pregnancies. The importance of three consecutive losses is significant. There is approximately a 15–20 percent chance that a woman may lose any pregnancy, without any apparent problem existing. These women usually go on to have uneventful future pregnancies and deliveries. Just as there is a certain probability of a woman losing a single pregnancy, there is a certain random chance that two fetal losses may occur one after the other. But if three pregnancies are lost consecutively, then there is a very real possibility of there being something wrong. A woman who has miscarried once or twice need not necessarily be evaluated for a problem. However, the loss of three pregnancies indicates and justifies a medical evaluation. And more recent data suggest that it is appropriate to evaluate a couple after two consecutive miscarriages. (See Chapter 7.)

The inability to conceive may occur after you have had a child or without your ever having been pregnant before. These two possibilities are described by different terms. *Primary infertility* is infertility without any preexisting pregnancies. *Secondary infertility* is infertility following one or more pregnancies. In the case of secondary infertility, the couple has already demonstrated the ability to produce a child: the basic apparatus is present and capable of working at least once. In primary infertility, the couple has never produced a child. The basic reproductive apparatus has never been shown to work at all. Statistically, primary and secondary infertility each have different causes, though generally the same problems must be considered in each case.

Infertility is a symptom and not a specific disease. It is a manifestation of a problem that exists within a couple. The problem may be within the man or the woman, or both. Infertility is unique in that regardless of which individual may have the problem leading to infertility, the couple, rather than the individual, is affected.

Approximately 15 percent or more of the couples of reproductive age in the United States are infertile. Of these, approximately 40 percent have infertility of male origin and 50 percent of female origin. Previous estimates had been that the remaining 10 percent of infertile couples had infertility of undetermined cause. This last category refers to couples who have had a complete infertility evaluation, and no reason for infertility could be determined. It does not mean that these patients did not have a problem, but that the specialty of reproductive medicine could not determine what their problem was. In order to adequately treat a couple, we must find the cause of their infertility. If we cannot determine the cause, we cannot institute appropriate treatment. Thus, that group with unexplained infertility represents an area of particular frustration for both the couple and the physician. With the advances in reproductive medicine, the percentage of couples with unexplained infertility has gradually decreased; a recent estimate was put at approximately 3.5 percent. This means that as the science of reproductive medicine gradually evolves, we are finding more with diagnosable problems and fewer couples with "unexplained infertility." As more problems can be diagnosed more couples can be successfully treated. The result is more pregnancies for those patients who desire them.

In order to understand how pregnancy occurs normally, and therefore how it can fail to occur in an infertile couple, you first

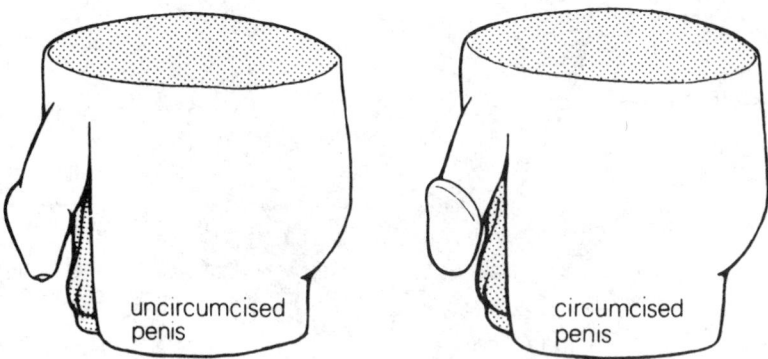

uncircumcised
penis

circumcised
penis

Figure 1.1a *External genitalia.*

need to know a bit about the anatomy of both the normal male and female.

MALE ANATOMY

Let us begin with the anatomy of the man. The male sex organs consist of a *penis* and two *testes*, sometimes referred to as *testicles*, enclosed within a pouch of skin and fibrous tissue called the *scrotum*. The *testes* are a source of sperm cells and hormones, most notably *testosterone*. Testosterone is a chemical substance responsible for the shape and characteristics of the male body, such as the texture of skin, hair distribution, voice quality, etc. The testes are connected to the penis by a system of tubes. The testis itself is composed of multiple lobules, each one containing the *seminiferous tubules*, the apparatus necessary to produce many sperm cells. The lobules are connected to small channels which all empty into larger ducts, and finally into a structure called the *epididymis*. The epididymis is a somewhat coiled, tubular structure which then directly joins the *vas deferens*, a rather straight, tubular structure. The vas deferens from each testis goes up in the scrotum and enters the penis within the

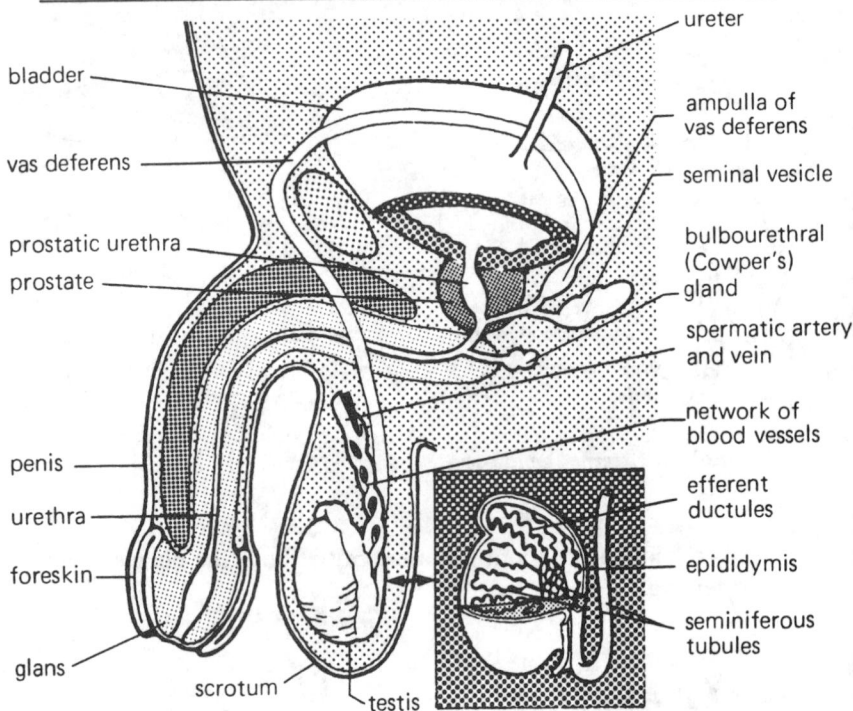

Figure 1.1b *Internal genitalia (cross-section schematic view).*

abdomen. The penis has a channel within it called the *urethra*. It is through the urethra that sperm is released and that urine is excreted. The vas deferens joins the urethra by passing through the *ejaculatory ducts* and the *prostate gland.* Sperm is produced within the seminiferous tubules of the testis by a process known as *spermatogenesis.* The sperm enters the network of tubules and eventually gains access to the epididymis. It is within this chamberlike area that further maturation and development of the sperm cells takes place. Within the epididymis, sperm cells are moved along by a series of muscular contractions of the tube known as *peristalsis.* From the epididymis the sperm enters the vas deferens and travels up to the area of the prostate. At the point of junction of the vas deferens and the urethra, a small, convoluted, saclike area called the *seminal vesicle* is found. The sperm produced and carried up through the vas deferens is stored near the seminal vesicle. The stored sperm then enters the urethra where secretions from the seminal vesicle and the prostate are added. The sperm and secretions travel along the urethra and leave the body through the tip of the penis (Figures 1.1a and 1.1b).

Ejaculation, the release of sperm at the time of orgasm, occurs when the seminal fluid reaches the area of the urethra that is within the prostate. The fluid and sperm cells are propelled forward by the contractions of the muscles within the penis. The tip of the penis is very sensitive to touch and other forms of stimulation. Its sensitivity and behavior are very much like that of the female clitoris. Upon stimulation, a number of nerve pathways are activated and a muscular ring around the opening of the bladder is caused to close, thereby preventing the sperm from entering the bladder. Such a backward release of sperm into the bladder rather than being emitted through the penis is called *retrograde ejaculation.*

Certain drugs, such as antidepressants and anti–high blood pressure medications, may diminish the ability of the muscular ring around the opening of the bladder to contract and thereby allow retrograde ejaculation to occur. If the sperm goes backward into the bladder, a very small number of sperm cells may be released through the penis and infertility may result.

The first part of the ejaculate emitted from the penis is rich in sperm while the last part is fluid and contains few sperm cells. If the man has a very low sperm count and a high semen volume it is possible to artificially raise the concentration of his ejaculate by discarding the second, sperm-poor portion and using only the first, highly concentrated portion for the purpose of producing a pregnancy.

FEMALE ANATOMY

A woman's reproductive organs can arbitrarily be divided into two areas (Figures 1.2a and 1.2b), external organs or *external genitalia* and internal organs or *internal genitalia.*

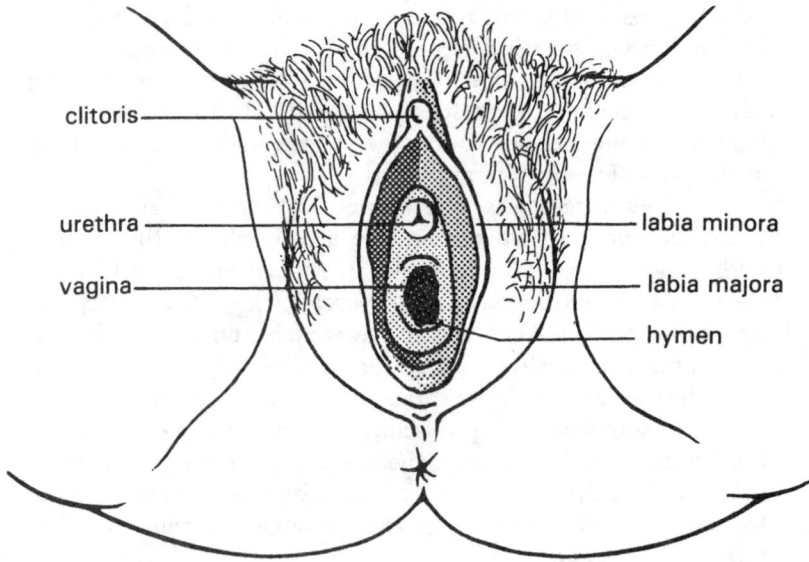

Figure 1.2a *External genitalia.*

The external genitalia consist of a double set of liplike structures surrounding the vagina. The inner lips on either side of the vagina are called the *labia minora.* Outside the labia minora are larger liplike structures called the *labia majora.* The labia minora connect above the vagina and cover a small, highly sensitive erectile structure called the *clitoris.*

The clitoris has many sensory nerve endings and is exquisitely sensitive to touch and stimulation. Part of its response to stimulation is enlargement and the increase of secretions within the vagina. Upon stimulation the clitoris becomes filled with blood and somewhat erect. At this time it appears very much like a miniature penis. Embryologically, it derives from the same area in the fetus as does the tip of the penis. Just below the clitoris is a small opening called the *urethral meatus* through which a woman urinates. Below this opening is the *vaginal canal.*

The internal genitalia are composed of the *vagina, cervix,*

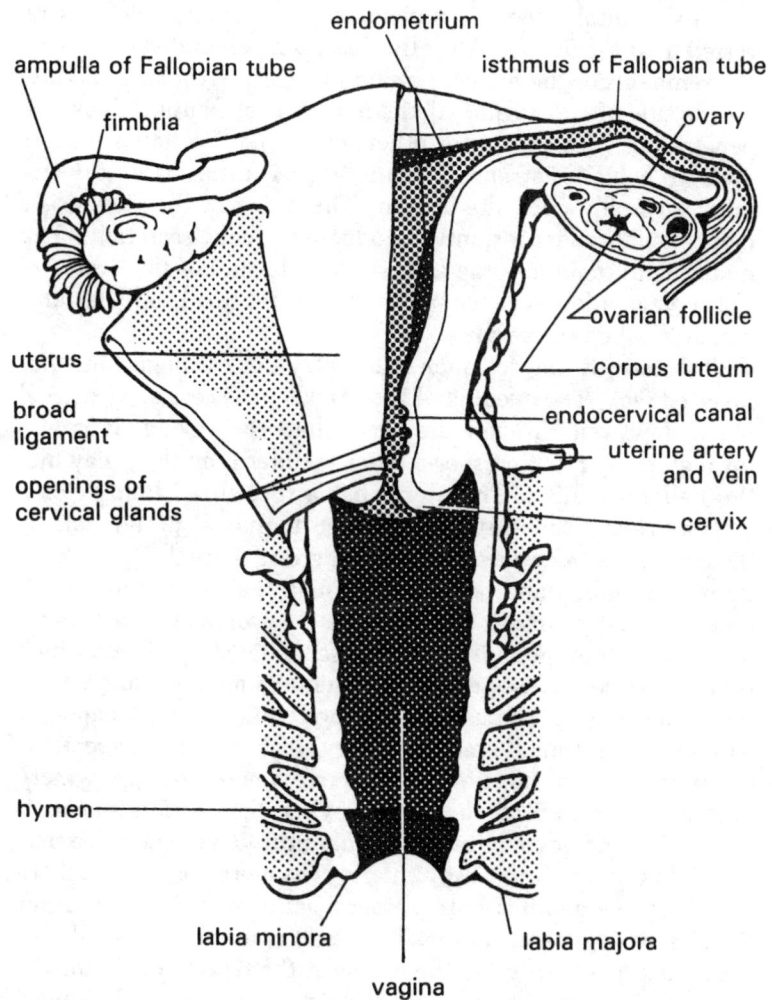

Figure 1.2b *Internal genitalia (schematic view).*

uterus, Fallopian tubes, and *ovaries.* The vagina is a long, tube-like structure connecting the uterus with the outer world by way of the external genitalia. At the junction of the vagina with the external genitalia there is a membrane of varying thickness referred to as the *hymen.* After this has been penetrated or broken, the remnants of the hymen remain as small, irregular structures on the side of the vagina. If the hymen is of unusual thickness, penetration with a penis or other means may be impossible. In order to achieve entrance into the vagina in this case, a doctor must surgically open the hymen. The lining of the vagina is a moist membrane constantly producing mucus secretion. This mucus fluid maintains the soft, slippery texture of the tissue.

The vagina joins the *womb* or uterus at a small, circular area which is called the cervix.

The uterus is shaped much like a very thick walled, muscular inverted sack. The opening of the "sack" is the cervix. Menstrual blood flows out through the cervix into the vagina. It is also through the cervix that sperm enter the uterus on their way into the Fallopian tubes. The uterus has a specialized lining called *endometrium.* This tissue responds to hormonal production by the ovary. At times the endometrium grows quite thick. At other times it crumbles and pours out through the cervix into the vagina. When it pours out it is known as the woman's *period, menses,* or *menstrual flow.* The cervix itself is lined by glands which produce mucus. The quality and volume of mucus changes with the woman's cycle. Discussion of the cycle will occur in Chapter 2. At most times a small amount of very thick mucus is present. At the time of ovulation, however, a large amount of very watery mucus is produced by the cervix. When the cervical mucus is very thick and present in small quantities it acts as a barrier, preventing sperm from easily entering the uterus. But when there is more mucus and it is watery, sperm can swim through it rather than becoming trapped in it. The result is that the cervical mucus favors sperm entering the uterus at the time of ovulation.

The uterus is positioned within the woman's pelvis. It is most frequently tilted forward, bending toward the front of the woman's abdomen. This uterus is described as being *anteverted* and *anteflexed.* The uterus may be tilted backward so that it is bend-

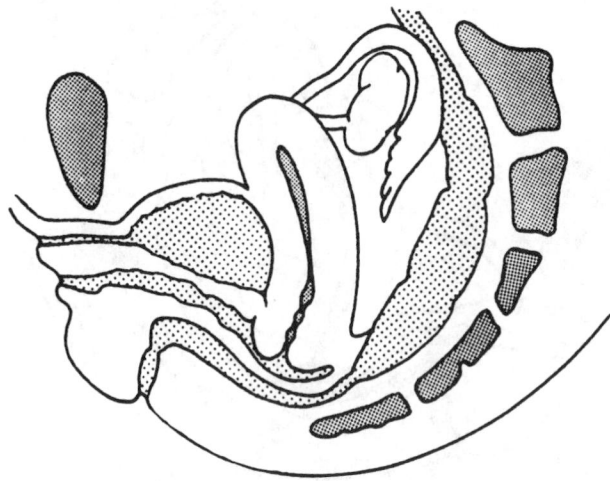

Figure 1.3 *An anteverted or normally positioned uterus.*

ing in the direction of the woman's back. In this case the uterus is described as being *retroverted* and *retroflexed*. The common term for this last condition is a *tipped uterus*. A uterus which is tilted forward is more common than a uterus which is tilted backward. Because something is less common does not mean that it is abnormal. If most people had brown eyes and one person had blue eyes, saying that you had blue eyes would not mean that you had anything wrong with you. It would simply be a way of describing you. Telling a woman that she has a tipped uterus is simply a way of describing the position of her uterus but by itself does not imply that there is anything wrong with it. Approximately 80 percent of women have an anteverted uterus and 20 percent have a retroverted uterus (Figures 1.3 and 1.4).

Projecting one off each side of the body of the uterus are two tubes. These structures, called the Fallopian tubes or *oviducts,* form the passages through which the egg is conducted from the ovary into the uterus. The Fallopian tubes are relatively long structures with specialized funnel-shaped, mobile areas at their

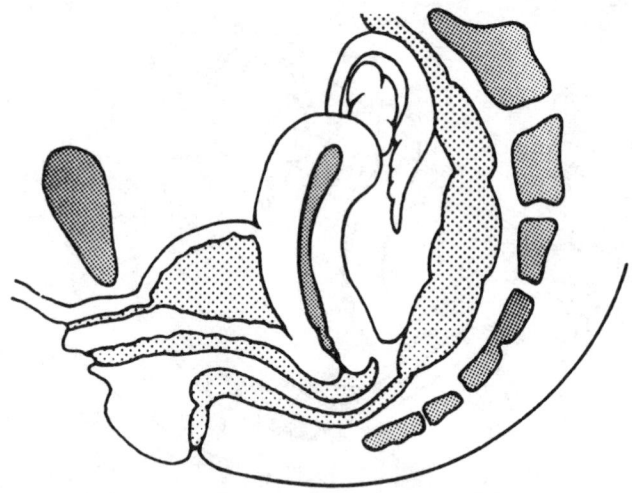

Figure 1.4 *Retroverted or tipped uterus.*

outer ends. The funnel-shaped area is called the *fimbria* and is specially designed to pick up eggs. The Fallopian tube itself is a muscular, highly movable tubular structure capable of very coordinated movement. Its lining is folded and lined with microscopic hairlike projections called *cilia*, which together are capable of creating highly coordinated movements. The tubal lining, called the *endosalpinx*, is also capable of producing a fluid that can act as a nutritive medium for the egg. The fertilized egg is conducted down the oviduct by the contractions of its muscular wall and by the beating of the cilia.

The ovaries are structures the size and shape of an olive just under the Fallopian tubes and to the side of the body of the uterus. The ovaries release an *ovum* (egg) at the time of ovulation. Ovaries are also the source of hormones such as *estrogen* and *progesterone*. At the time of ovulation the ovary releases an egg which is picked up by the fimbria. The egg is conducted through the internal channel of the Fallopian tube to approximately the middle third of the tube. If the man and woman make love at the time of ovulation, the sperm will mix with the watery cervical mucus and swim through the cervix into the uterine cavity. The sperm will be actively conducted through the uterine cavity into the Fallopian tubes. A sperm cell and the egg which was released will unite by a process called *fertilization*. The fertilized egg then moves through the Fallopian tube into the uterine cavity where it attaches to the uterine lining. This newly fertilized egg grows into an embryo, a fetus, and, later, a baby.

WHEN SHOULD A COUPLE BE EVALUATED?

The next problem that must be reviewed is at what point a couple should decide that they have an infertility problem. At what point should a couple seek the advice of a physician for the problems of infertility? The definition of infertility specifies that a couple should have regular sexual relations for at least one year without conception. As mentioned earlier, regular sexual relations means making love every other day around ovulation time, or every other day throughout the cycle, every month for twelve months. At this point in our discussion it may not be obvious as to how the determination of ovulation time is made. This will be discussed at length in Chapter 5. This "one-year period" applies whether or not the couple has previously achieved pregnancy.

If, on the other hand, the couple has achieved pregnancy and two consecutive pregnancies have ended spontaneously without the birth of a live child, then that too is an indication to seek medical help. As with anything, these are only guidelines, not absolute rules. They are set up so that those who have the greatest need may get attention while those couples with the greatest probability of having no problem will not undertake an unnecessary infertility investigation.

As said earlier, these are not absolute rules and must be tempered by the judgment of your doctor. It is apparent that if on initial review of the couple's history, it can be seen that the man is unable to ejaculate, that is, release semen from his penis on orgasm, or it is unlikely that the woman is ovulating at all, there would be nothing gained by waiting a full year before beginning an evaluation.

EVALUATION: COST AND DISCOMFORT

People are often afraid that an evaluation will be painful, long in duration, and extremely costly. This is usually not the case. The period of time for evaluation depends upon the kinds of problems the studies find. Usually, the time frame is several weeks to months. The cost varies tremendously but if finances are a problem, infertility clinics usually are available in most areas. Discomfort is a very private matter. What is tolerable to one person may be agony to another. Nevertheless, it is my experience that in the hands of an experienced practitioner, the infertility workup can take place with a minimal degree of discomfort. I do not say this as a disinterested third party, but as a human being strongly involved in the feelings of my patients. I could not bring myself to cause repeated or significant discomfort to anyone.

Now that the basics have been presented, the next step is to see how everything fits together for the production of a pregnancy.

CHAPTER 2

Baby Production: The Way It Should Work

AT FIRST it appears that producing a child is really not terribly difficult. All that is required is that one healthy sperm and a healthy egg, an ovum, be in the same place at the same time so that the two can unite. The resulting fertilized ovum then must be kept in a protected area for approximately forty weeks and given proper nourishment and room to grow. Any interruption in this basic scheme that prevents the egg and sperm from uniting or that makes it impossible for the fertilized egg to develop will result in infertility. The ways this scheme can be interrupted are many. Before you can understand what can go wrong, you must first understand what happens when things work properly.

AN OVERVIEW

After a normal menstrual flow, several eggs within the woman's ovary begin to develop. Soon, one of these developing eggs matures more than the rest and, in approximately fourteen days after the onset of menstrual flow, this mature egg pops out of the surface of the ovary. This is known as *ovulation*. A specialized, funnel-shaped structure at the end of the Fallopian tube called the fimbria will pick up this egg and the lining of the tube will move the egg down the oviduct to approximately the middle third of the tube. If a couple makes love at this time, sperm released by the penis are placed within the vagina next to the

17

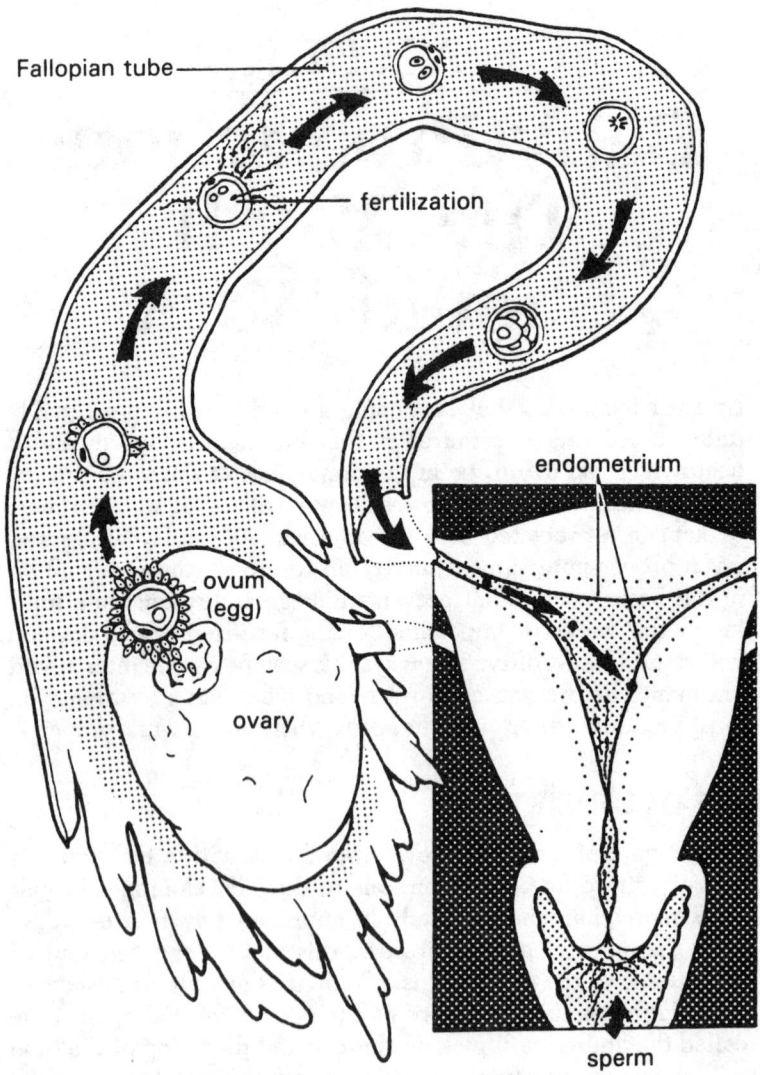

Figure 2.1 *Ovulation and fertilization.*

cervix (the opening of the womb). The sperm cells swim through the cervical mucus at the opening of the uterus (the womb) and are carried into the cavity of the uterus and up into the Fallopian tube. This trip takes only about ten to twenty minutes. The sperm and the egg are now in the same place and, by random movement, we hope that one sperm cell will meet this egg and the two will unite, causing fertilization. The fertilized egg now begins to move down the tube again, toward the uterus. It crosses into the uterine cavity, the space within the uterus, and adheres to the lining of this cavity. This is called *implantation.* The tissue lining the wall of the uterus is very thick, filled with blood vessels, and capable of delivering nourishment to this newly fertilized egg. The fertilized egg quickly develops and progresses into an embryo, eventually a fetus, and then a new human being. As time passes, the *placenta,* a specialized organ within the uterine cavity connecting the fetus to the mother, will grow, providing nutrition and respiration to the developing fetus.

A MORE DETAILED VIEW

This discussion started by simply saying that ovulation (the release of an egg) occurred, but ovulation does not just happen without preparation. Eggs do not just develop in the ovary, mature, and pop out of the surface without an appropriate stimulus. Furthermore, the lining of the uterus has to be carefully prepared so that the fertilized egg can implant onto it. The body requires some kind of synchronized mechanism to control the release of the egg and the development of the lining of the uterus so that when the egg finally gets to the uterine cavity, the lining is prepared to support it for many weeks in its development toward becoming a human being. This is how it happens.

Hormonal Stimulus

In the floor of the brain is a gland called the *pituitary gland.* This is sometimes called the "master gland" because it controls the functioning of many other glands distributed throughout the body. Just above the pituitary is a section of the brain called the *hypothalamus,* which in turn controls the pituitary gland and is itself controlled by higher centers of the brain. The result is a neurological system in which components are interconnected like the wires of a vast telephone network. Though the pituitary gland produces many hormones, at this moment we are interested only in two, one called *FSH,* follicle-stimulating hormone, and the other, *LH,* luteinizing hormone. FSH and LH are released into the bloodstream and when they reach the ovary they stimulate it so that *estrogen* is produced and several eggs begin to ripen. The estrogen produced by the ovary enters the blood and is distributed throughout the body. It is estrogen that is important in determining the shape of the female's body, the development of her breasts, the texture of her skin, the development and texture of her hair, and even the secretions within her vagina. Estrogen also stimulates the lining of the uterus to grow in a very specific manner, (that is, to proliferate and grow thicker).

The release of FSH and LH from the pituitary gland is controlled by and generally influenced by the hypothalamus. The hypothalamus secretes a protein called *gonadotropin-releasing hormone, GnRH,* which is carried down into the pituitary and acts upon the cells that produce and release FSH and LH. GnRH is not released in a constant fashion but in small bursts occurring approximately six minutes every sixty to ninety minutes. It is this slow, repetitive stimulus of GnRH on the pituitary cells that is responsible for FSH and LH production and release.

These pituitary hormones enter the bloodstream and stimulate the ovary to produce estrogen. Estrogen, in turn, enters the bloodstream and is distributed throughout the body, returning to the pituitary. There it changes the effect that the repetitive pulsing release of GnRH has on the pituitary cells. When estrogen reaches a certain level in the bloodstream, the same repetitive GnRH signal that occurs throughout the cycle releases a large amount of FSH and LH from the pituitary. This massive release of FSH and LH—or LH surge, as it is called—causes the egg which is most mature to be released by the ovary, thus resulting in ovulation. (See Figures 2.2, 2.3a, 2.3b.)

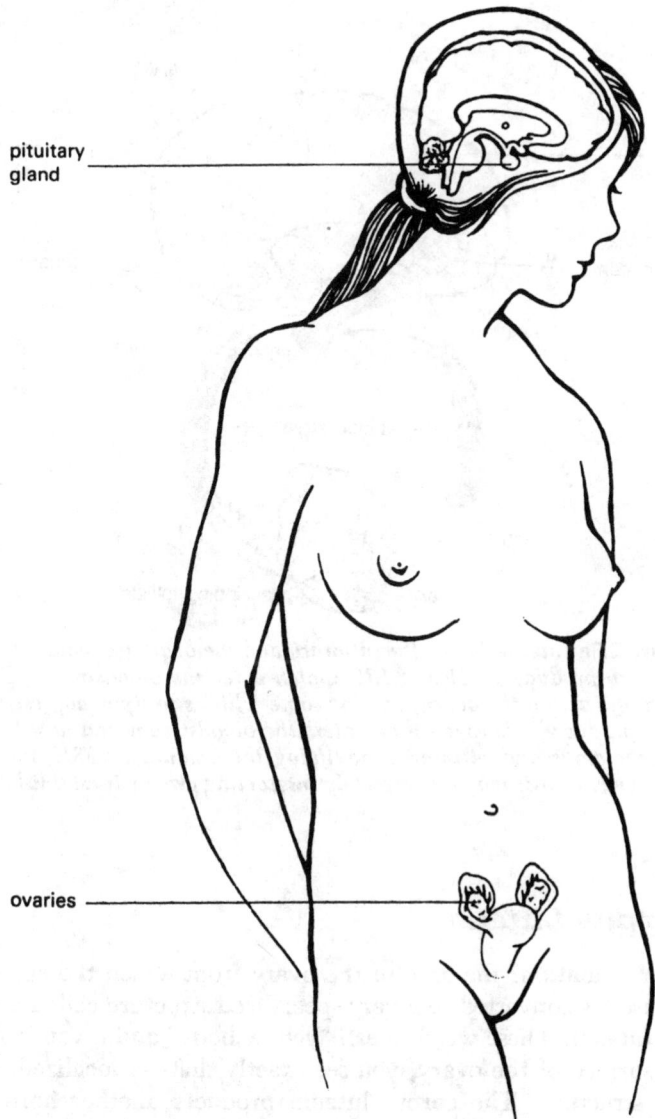

pituitary
gland

ovaries

Figure 2.2 *The location of the pituitary gland and the ovaries.*

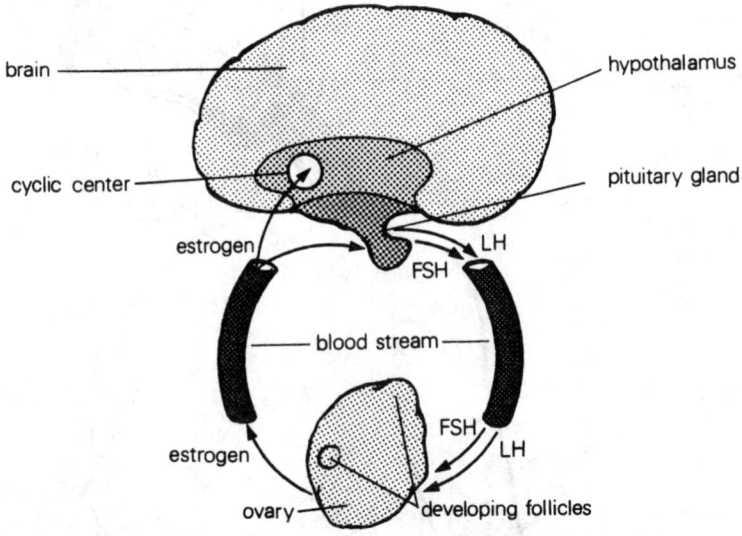

Figure 2.3a *Interaction of the pituitary and the ovary (schematic). The pituitary produces FSH and LH, which enter the bloodstream. These hormones act on the ovary, causing some follicles to ripen and estrogen to be produced. Estrogen then enters the bloodstream and acts on the hypothalamus and pituitary, modifying the amount of FSH and LH produced. In this way a completely interacting circuit is established.*

Corpus Luteum

After ovulation, the area of the ovary from which the egg was released is converted to a very specialized structure called a *corpus luteum*. These words mean "yellow body" and if you look at the surface of the ovary, you see exactly that—a localized, yellow structure. The corpus luteum produces another hormone called *progesterone*. Progesterone enters the circulatory system and, when it reaches the tissue lining the uterus, it causes a

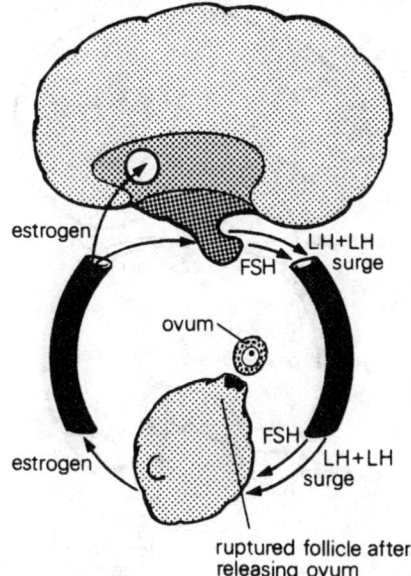

Figure 2.3b *In order for ovulation to occur, a sudden massive amount of LH must be released from the pituitary. When this happens a ripened follicle bursts and an ovum (egg) is released from the surface of the ovary. This massive release of LH producing ovulation is called the LH surge.*

change in the structure of the lining so that it can better provide support and nourishment to the newly fertilized egg. It takes approximately five days for the newly fertilized egg to reach the lining of the uterus. This ensures enough time for the uterine lining to develop the appropriate tissue which can best keep this developing human being alive. (See Figure 2.3c.)

And so the same mechanisms that allow for the development of an egg and its release from the surface of the ovary also allow for the preparation of the lining of the uterus to properly accept and maintain the fertilized egg.

The corpus luteum, the yellow body, may be thought of as a progesterone-producing factory within the surface of the ovary. This progesterone factory is controlled by the pituitary gland

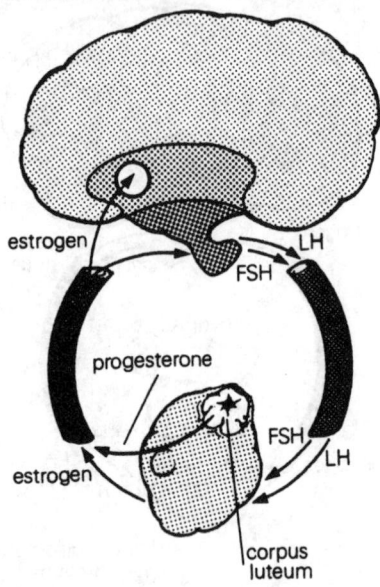

Figure 2.3c *After ovulation, the corpus luteum, found on the site of the ruptured follicle, produces progesterone.*

and, if pregnancy does not occur, the factory fails and shuts off after fourteen days of functioning. Progesterone production stops and the uterine lining can no longer be maintained in its preparatory state. With the end of progesterone production the uterine lining crumbles and sloughs. The entire lining is shed over a three- to five-day interval and when it flows out through the cervix and into the vagina it is recognized as the woman's menstrual period.

For pregnancy to occur, the lining of the uterus must be maintained by progesterone for longer than the usual fourteen-day life of the corpus luteum. Then, if an egg is fertilized and pregnancy does occur, the newly developing placental tissue takes control of the corpus luteum and keeps it functioning into the early weeks of pregnancy.

Menstrual Cycle

A woman normally releases an egg from her ovary about once a month. If she does not become pregnant she will get her menstrual flow fourteen days after ovulation. The interval of time from the first day of bleeding in one month to the first day of bleeding in the next month is referred to as the menstrual cycle. The days of the menstrual cycle are numbered consecutively from the first day of vaginal bleeding. The first day of the menstrual flow is always called cycle day one regardless of what the calendar date might be. If your period began on August 20, then August 20 was cycle day one of that menstrual cycle.

The most common length of a menstrual cycle is twenty-eight days, with ovulation occurring on cycle day fourteen. Estrogen is produced by the ovary during the entire menstrual cycle but progesterone is produced only from ovulation to just before the onset of menses (cycle day fourteen to twenty-eight).

When estrogen acts alone on the uterine lining it produces a characteristic tissue called *proliferative endometrium*. After ovulation, when, in addition to the estrogen, progesterone is produced by the corpus luteum, the uterine lining is converted to *secretory endometrium*. It is secretory endometrium that is prepared to receive and nourish the newly fertilized egg. The secretory endometrium changes in structure each day under the influence of progesterone. The changes are so precise and predictable that it is possible to look at the microscopic structure of a piece of secretory endometrium and to know how many days earlier ovulation occurred. (See Figure 2.4.)

For the sake of further discussion, the first half of the menstrual cycle, when estrogen alone is being produced, is called the *proliferative phase* of the cycle. The second half of the cycle is called the *secretory phase*. The secretory phase is fixed at fourteen days, but the proliferative phase can vary in length from woman to woman, or even in the same woman from cycle to cycle. If a woman has a twenty-eight–day menstrual cycle she has a fourteen-day proliferative phase, ovulates on cycle day fourteen, and has a fourteen-day secretory phase. If her cycle is

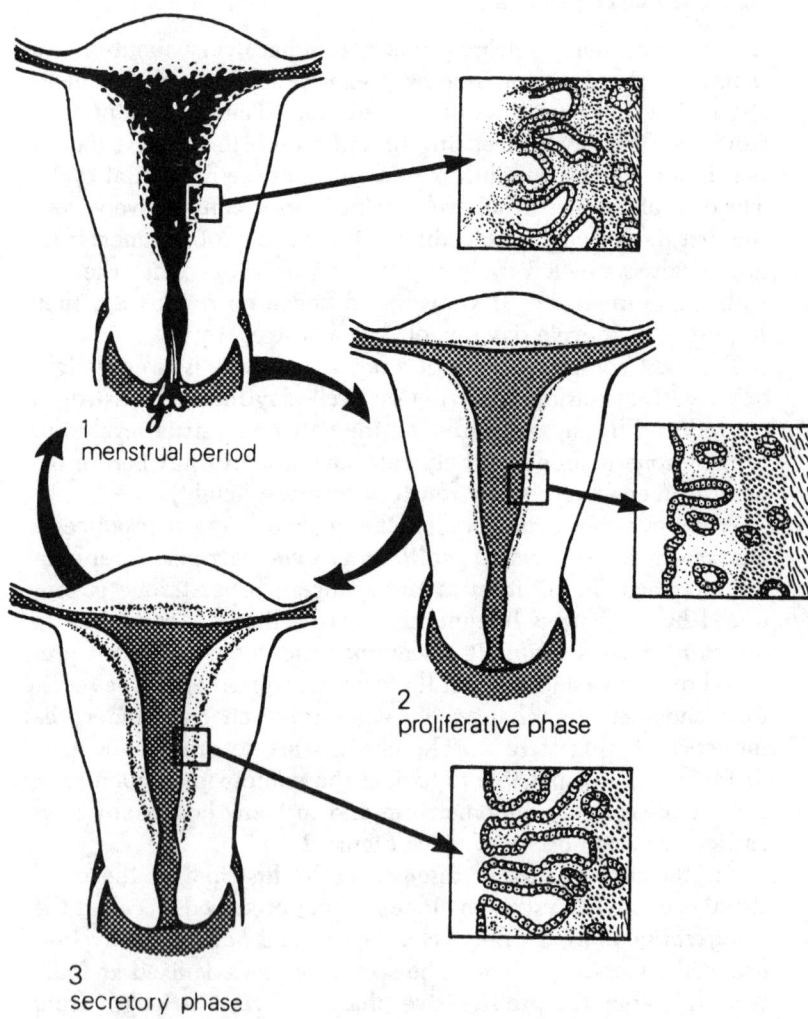

Figure 2.4 *Phases of the menstrual cycle. The lining of the uterus grows and changes during the menstrual cycle. During the proliferative phase it grows and thickens. In the secretory phase it is readied to receive a fertilized egg. If pregnancy does not occur, the lining crumbles and is seen as the woman's menstrual flow.*

thirty days in length, the first half of her cycle is sixteen days long with ovulation occurring on cycle day sixteen. Similarly, if a woman has a twenty-five–day cycle, that means that the proliferative phase is eleven days long and that ovulation occurs on cycle day eleven. In women who have cycles of varying lengths, it is always the first half of the cycle that varies in duration while the second half remains fixed. Since ovulation occurs at the end of the proliferative phase and may vary in length, it may be difficult to determine exactly when ovulation occurs in a woman with a variable cycle while that cycle is occurring. However, when menses occur, all the woman has to do to determine when the egg was released is to count back fourteen days. Unfortunately, this is after the fact, and this method is of less than ideal help during the cycles that a couple is attempting pregnancy. (See Figure 2.5.)

Fertilization

Fertilization is a random thing. Though that statement sounds like a 1938 song title, it has a great deal of significance. A sperm and an egg may both be in the same area of the tube at the same time. The two meet by random movement, or dumb luck, if you will. As if to increase the chances of fertilization, nature allows not one but hundreds of thousands of sperm cells to arrive in the tube in the area of the egg. The greater the number of sperm around the egg, the greater the chance of one of those sperm meeting and fertilizing that egg. Still, even if a couple makes love on the day before, the day of, and the day after ovulation, pregnancy usually does not occur during the first cycle. It can take up to one year, twelve cycles of regular sexual activity or more, for a normal couple to achieve a pregnancy.

These are the basic mechanisms of ovulation and fertilization. In the next chapter I discuss some of the errors and myths commonly accepted as truth.

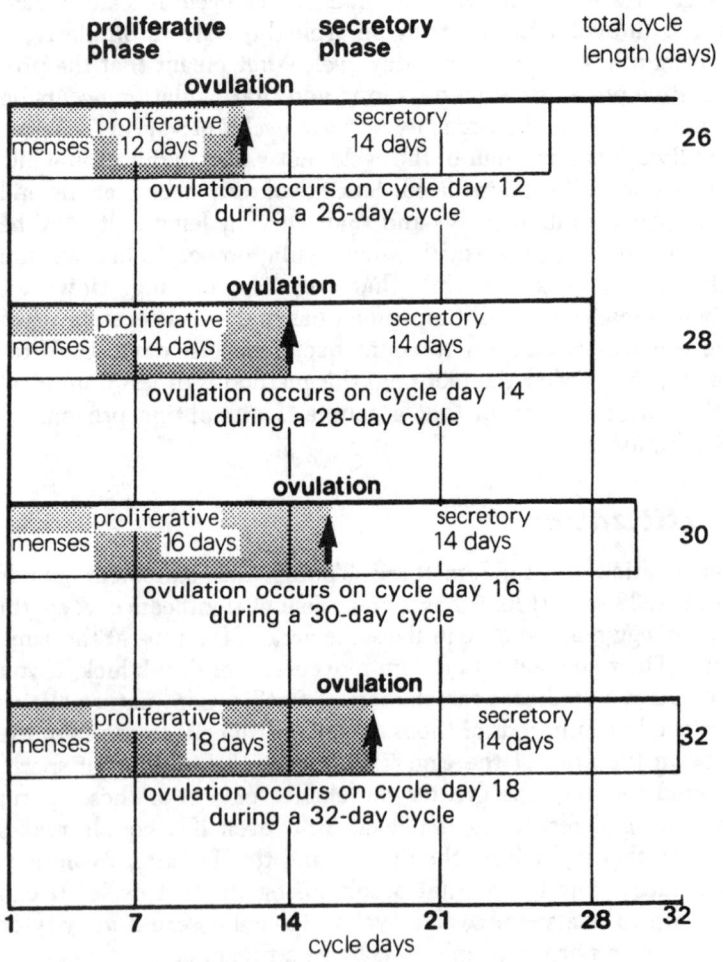

Figure 2.5 *Numbering the days of the menstrual cycle. The first day of a woman's menstrual period (menses) is called cycle day one. The second half of the menstrual cycle, the secretory phase, is fixed at fourteen days in length, while the first half, the proliferative phase, varies with the length of the cycle. Ovulation occurs at the end of the proliferative phase.*

By subtracting fourteen from the total number of days of the menstrual cycle, one gets the day of theoretical ovulation.

CHAPTER 3

Myths, Misconceptions, and Misinformation

Now THAT I have reviewed the basic mechanisms involved in ovulation and the establishment of pregnancy, I will discuss some of the fables and misinformation regarding human reproduction. Some of these statements will seem ridiculous. Nevertheless, it is important to explore them to underline their inaccuracy and to emphasize the general concepts presented thus far.

Pregnancy always occurs immediately if intercourse has occurred at ovulation time.

The meeting of the sperm and the egg occurs by random movement. Thus, even though a man and a woman may have intercourse at the right time of the woman's cycle and sperm cells may enter the female reproductive tract, it does not necessarily follow that a sperm and an egg will actually meet. Since fertilization takes place by the random meeting of the sperm and the egg, a number of attempts are necessary for an egg to become fertilized. Given enough tries, over enough cycles, the chances that fertilization will take place are generally good. Approximately 25 percent of couples attempting pregnancy will achieve it within one month. Approximately 80 percent of couples will conceive within one year's time. It is because of this that couples are usually not investigated for infertility unless they have attempted pregnancy with regular sexual relations for twelve cycles and have failed to conceive. Both theory and statistics show that pregnancy usually does not occur right away even if sexual activity was perfectly timed.

In summary—failing to achieve conception after a single cycle is not a sign of a problem.

Ovulation alternates from one ovary one month to the opposite ovary the next month.

Ovulation does not alternate from one ovary to the other. Over the course of the year each ovary appears to ovulate approximately an equal number of times, but the pattern is random rather than alternating. At the beginning of a cycle it is impossible to predict which ovary will be the one to release an egg. Ovulation may occur from the right ovary one month but the following month the chances are just as great that ovulation will occur from the right ovary again as from the left one.

The picture becomes more complicated because it is not always the tube on the same side as the ovulating ovary that picks up the egg. There are women who had only one tube and one ovary, each on opposite sides, who have achieved pregnancy. What appears to have happened is that the egg was released by the ovary and the tube on the opposite side crossed over to pick it up. These are unusual cases. In the vast majority of women, the tube on the same side picks up the freshly released egg.

There is no way to predict which ovary will release an egg during any given cycle or even to know with certainty which tube will pick up the egg.

Menses indicate ovulation has occurred.

Another way of stating this widely held chestnut is by saying, "If you had a period, you know you have ovulated." Both of these statements are frequently made and both are quite false. Menses indicate only that the lining of the uterus has been partially or completely shed. This usually happens fourteen days after an ovulation if pregnancy has not occurred. However, if ovulation fails to occur, the lining of the uterus may continue to grow as a proliferative endometrium. After several weeks the lining becomes thicker and progressively more brittle. A point is reached where, like piling too many building blocks one on top of the other, the lining outgrows its structural support and begins to crumble. At this time the tissue breaks off and flows out of the cervix into the vagina and appears very much like the menses following an ovulation. In this case, however, the bleeding that occurs does not follow an ovulation. This is called nonovulatory or *anovulatory bleeding*.

Anovulatory bleeding, since it is the result of random breaking and sloughing of tissue, may produce almost any kind of menstrual pattern. A woman may experience a menstrual flow that appears to be normal both in amount and duration or she may experience extremely light or extremely heavy vaginal bleeding. Bleeding may go on for several hours or may continue for weeks or months. The point is that the presence of vaginal bleeding, or menses, does not necessarily mean that ovulation has occurred.

After the age of thirty, you had better not try to get pregnant because the chances of an abnormal child are very, very high.

With increasing age the chances of a woman delivering an abnormal child increase slightly. After the age of thirty-five, however, with each increasing year thereafter, the chances of an abnormal newborn increase significantly. The chances of a complication occurring to the mother during pregnancy also increase year by year after the age of thirty-five. During the same period of time a woman's spontaneous fertility seems to decrease. This almost seems to be an inborn protective mechanism for the mother, child, and species: fetal and maternal complications increase while spontaneous female fertility decreases after the age of thirty-five. Though this has been supported by numerous studies, recent investigation has questioned these findings. It may be the case that the increase in fetal abnormality and maternal risk may be much less than initially anticipated. Only further studies by other investigators can confirm this.

It has now become possible to obtain information about the unborn baby. While in the uterus, the fetus floats in a waterlike environment called the *amniotic fluid*. It sheds cells and body chemicals into this liquid world. By inserting a long hypodermic needle through the abdomen and the uterus into the amniotic fluid, some of this material can be withdrawn and tests performed. The procedure of sampling the amniotic fluid is called *amniocentesis* and is usually done between the fourteenth and sixteenth week of pregnancy. One of the most common and significant tests done is the genetic study which can diagnose certain abnormalities such as *Down syndrome*, previously known as mongolism. (See Figure 3.1.)

By utilizing the information obtained from the amniotic fluid studies it is possible to tell a couple whether or not some of the disorders found in the children of older mothers exist in the unborn child. If such a problem is discovered, the couple may elect to end the pregnancy and thereby prevent the birth of an abnormal child. Using such an approach, the risk of a mother above the age of thirty-five having an abnormal child can be sharply reduced.

Based on current information, telling a woman between the ages of thirty and thirty-four not to consider childbearing would be overcautious and unfortunate. However, considering childbearing after the age of thirty-five deserves a significant amount of thought. (See Chapter 13.)

If you are frigid you cannot conceive.

Failing to be able to be sexually aroused rarely has a direct effect on being able to become pregnant. If frigidity results in a decreased frequency of sexual relations, then pregnancy becomes more difficult because there is less sexual exposure, not because of frigidity itself. If the frigidity is a result of a structural problem within the woman's vagina or of certain hormonal deficiencies, then these problems may in turn interfere with fertility. But the failure to be sexually stimulated and aroused in no way prevents ovulation and the ultimate union of a sperm and an egg. Though sexual arousal and satisfaction make coital activity more gratifying, they are not necessary to produce a child.

A "tipped uterus" makes it difficult to become pregnant.

Some years ago this was a widely held belief both among phy-

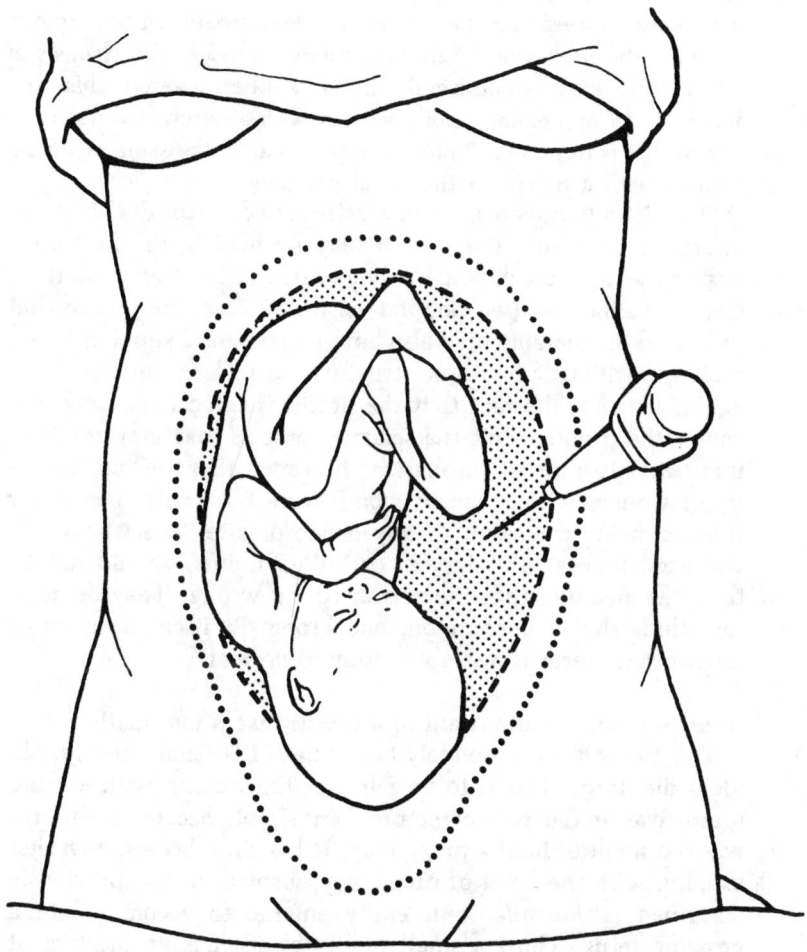

Figure 3.1 *Amniocentesis: the removal of some of the amniotic fluid to evaluate the condition of the fetus.*

sicians and the interested general public. It was felt that if the uterus was tipped backward it would be more difficult for sperm to enter the uterus and Fallopian tubes, therefore the chances of conception were diminished. Later studies showed that the incidence of pregnancy among women with a retroverted uterus (a womb that is tipped backward) is approximately the same as among women with a uterus in the usual position.

Occasionally a woman with a retroverted uterus does have an infertility problem. The womb may be held in the backward position as a result of some pelvic scarring, be it endometriosis or pelvic adhesions (see Chapter 4). In this case, the process that produced the scarring may also have scarred the Fallopian tubes, making it difficult for these structures to pick up an egg. Here again, it is not the fact that the uterus is tilted backward that causes the problem but the scarring process that may result in infertility. It must be emphasized however, that the vast majority of women with a tipped womb were born with one rather than its being the result of any pelvic disease. The words "retroverted uterus" or "tipped" or "tilted uterus" should not be taken as meaning that there is anything wrong. They describe something that is uncommon, not wrong. By itself, a tipped or retroverted uterus is just a variation of normal.

Infertility may be the result of a uterus that is too small.

This too was once a widely held belief. Like many things, old ideas die hard. It used to be felt that the woman with a small uterus was unable to become pregnant simply because the uterus was too small to hold a pregnancy. It has since been shown that usually, with the onset of pregnancy, a small uterus, previously described as *juvenile,* will easily enlarge to accommodate a growing fetus. Thus, a small uterus by itself is an insufficient reason for infertility.

When a couple has an infertility problem it is best for them to make love with the woman lying on her back with a pillow beneath her buttocks and for the man to assume a position on top of her. Upon completing relations, the woman should raise her legs against a wall and stay in this position for several hours.

Another variation of this is: **You are not getting pregnant because you are using the wrong position when making love.**

Unfortunately, there is no magic position that makes pregnancy significantly more likely. If the instructions given above were truly useful, then the best means of *contraception* would be to avoid the position described and for a woman to jump up and down after sex to dislodge the sperm. This particular means of contraception was practiced at the turn of the century but, unfortunately, with no demonstrable success.

At the time of ovulation, the cervix is surrounded by a large volume of very watery mucus. This is produced by the cervix and seems to act as an excellent medium to trap sperm cells and to aid them on their trip into the uterine cavity on their way to the Fallopian tube. Once sperm are deposited in the area of the cervix it takes only ten to twenty minutes for them to travel from the cervical mucus up to the Fallopian tube. This seems to be the case regardless of what positions are used during intercourse. Since the basic trip only takes ten to twenty minutes, suggesting that a woman place herself in a position to facilitate sperm movement into her reproductive tract and hold that position for several hours is illogical and unnecessary. A couple should have intercourse without using lubricants such as petroleum jelly, using whatever techniques they find pleasurable, and the woman should linger in bed for approximately thirty minutes after intercourse in any recumbent position she finds comfortable. In this way, ample opportunity is given for the sperm to enter the uterus and Fallopian tubes without the need for using uncomfortable and unnecessary positions.

If you want to get pregnant, go on a vacation.

This is a frequently heard suggestion, usually followed by a story of a friend, neighbor, or relative who had an infertility problem and then finally conceived following a vacation. If infertility is a symptom of an underlying problem influencing the reproductive system, then what can a vacation do? How can the stories be explained?

The explanation is fairly simple. Approximately 5 percent of infertile couples conceive without any treatment. This is the *spontaneous fertility rate* of infertile couples. In order to say that any treatment actually does something for a patient it must be shown to have a higher success rate than 5 percent—the pregnancy rate when no treatment is done. If a drug or operation is associated with a 5 percent pregnancy rate then we assume the treatment was of little of no help. On the other hand, if couples were given an unrelated therapy, such as having rocks taped to their armpits, a certain percentage, the same 5 percent, will conceive. Vacations fit into this last category. They may be enjoyable in themselves, but as a treatment for infertility they appear to be no more successful than doing nothing at all.

I have heard of infertile couples who adopt a child and then are able to have a child of their own. So, if you are having trouble getting pregnant, adopt first.

The pregnancy rate following adoption is the same as the rate when no treatment is given. Thus, adoption can be shown to do nothing to improve the chances of conception. The explanation is the same as just presented for the effect of vacations on infertility.

More important, adopting a child is indeed one approach to the treatment of infertility, but not in the way the above misconception suggests. Adoption is an end in itself, directly fulfilling the needs of a child and a couple. It must not be thought of as a means of inducing a pregnancy. With the increased use of contraception and the liberal use of abortion, the number of adoptable children is vastly reduced. In my opinion, these children should be considered for couples who in spite of treatment cannot conceive, and not as therapy to assist conception.

Infertility is usually a result of a problem with the woman.

This frequently stated observation is a wholesale slander leveled against women. It has resulted in needless grief and guilt and has actually prevented proper infertility evaluation by making some men unwilling to be studied. The precise numbers that one can present to counter this ridiculous statement may differ depending upon which studies one wishes to refer to. In general, male problems account for 40 percent of infertility, female problems account for 50 percent, and in 10 percent of couples no cause for infertility can be found. Thus, it is about as likely that infertility may be due to the man as to the woman.

More important, such a statement reflects a desire to assign fault to one member of a couple. It is not important who has the medical difficulty because it shows itself as a problem of the couple and not the individual, and must be approached as such. Furthermore, we do not usually feel guilty or make others feel guilty when they have medical problems. No one directs blame at an individual with an ulcer or gall stones. Infertility is a symptom of a medical dysfunction and should be approached no differently than any other medical problem.

These are some of the myths and misconceptions surrounding infertility. I certainly have not covered all of them, but it is clear that many widely held views are filled with inaccuracies. Having examined the inaccuracies, let us now progress to the next chapter, which will discuss the causes of infertility.

CHAPTER 4
The Causes of Infertility

BEFORE ONE can understand how to help a couple achieve a pregnancy, one must find the possible reasons that the couple has been unsuccessful up to this point. Chapter 2 described ovulation, the pathway the sperm follows in reaching the egg, fertilization, and the trip of the fertilized egg back to the protection of the uterus. A problem in any one of these steps, plus several not yet presented, will break the sequence of things and pregnancy will not occur. Since there are many steps in "baby production" and any one or more of them may go wrong resulting in infertility, the surprising thing is that anyone has been able to have a child at all.

For the purposes of this book, the causes of infertility will be grouped into six categories.

- Male factor—a problem in the male sex partner resulting in poor sperm production
- Female factor—a problem in the female sex partner stemming from lack of ovulation, a hormonal imbalance, and/or a structural abnormality
- Male—female interaction
- Psychological factor
- Genetic factor
- Infertility of undetermined cause

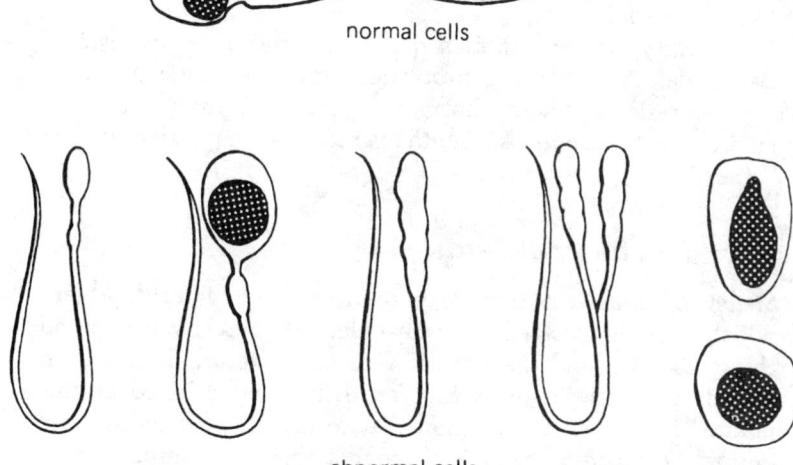

normal cells

abnormal cells

Figure 4.1. *Semen analysis. Not all the sperm cells produced are of normal shape. Both normal and abnormal forms are shown.*

EVALUATING THE MAN

To determine if *male factor infertility* is the problem, the doctor will do a microscopic examination of the man's sperm. This *semen analysis* may reveal that he is producing too few sperm to be able to fertilize a normal woman. It is not only the number of sperm cells that are produced that is important. The man must also produce an adequate percentage of motile (moving), normally shaped sperm cells, for it is only these cells that are capable of fertilizing an egg. It is possible for a man to have semen with an adequate number of sperm cells but with too few cells normal in both shape and motility to produce a pregnancy. Abnormalities in the semen specimen indicate the need for evaluation by a urologist specializing in male infertility. Hormonal studies, including thyroid and adrenal tests, and a physical examination looking for abnormalities of the testes should be done. (See Figure 4.1.)

Infertility problems in men may be a result of several categories of defects: structural problems, problems related to infection, genetic problems, hormonal problems, drug problems, environmental problems, and the general category referred to as "other."

Structural Problems

Structural problems that may result in male infertility vary widely. The *varicocele* is a grossly enlarged series of veins around the epididymis and the vas deferens of the testes. It results in infertility by mechanisms that are still being debated at this point. There is no explanation that seems to apply to all cases uniformly. In some cases it is thought that the unusually high temperature in the area of a varicocele may have a direct toxic effect upon the sperm-producing qualities of the testis. There are times when no adequate explanation seems to apply. Nevertheless, it seems that there is usually infertility when there is a varicocele. There is no correlation between the size of a varicocele and its effect on sperm production and sperm quality. The varicocele may be small and yet the effect on fertility may be great.

The doctor will examine the man while he bears down, very much as he would during a bowel movement, and feel the scrotum and testes. Because bearing down decreases the blood leaving these vessels, blood gathers in the swollen veins and they feel like pulsating worms. Surgery is the appropriate treatment.

Another structural abnormality may be the absence or obstruction of the vas deferens and/or the epididymis, the conduits of sperm from the testes to the penis. In this case, sperm is being produced by the testis but the route that it must travel to the penis is blocked. This may be a result of a congenital abnormality or may be a result of a purposeful surgical obstruction, such as following a vasectomy for sterilization.

The epididymis adds fructose to the semen. If the semen analysis shows no sperm and no fructose, these findings are consistent with the absence or the obstruction of the vas deferens or the epididymis. An obstruction of the vas deferens can usually be corrected by surgery. If no sperm are present but fructose can be found in the seminal fluid on masturbation, then there is a nonfunctioning testis but an open channel from the testes into the penis.

Another structural problem leading to infertility is *cryptorchidism*. In the embryo, the testes are in the abdomen and migrate into the scrotal sac by birth. Failure of the testes to descend into the scrotum is called cryptorchidism. Being in the abdomen severely affects the development of the testes and, if allowed to continue long enough, can prevent normal sperm development. If the doctor diagnoses an undescended testis, surgery to bring the testis into the scrotal sac should be considered. A biopsy of the testis will allow the patient and the doctor to judge his chances of producing a child in the future. A doctor can diagnose cryptorchidism simply by examining the scrotal sac to see whether or not testes are present. This clinical state must be differentiated from *anorchia*, where the man is born without testes. No testes are present either in the scrotum or in the abdomen. There is no way for a man with anorchia to father a child at this time.

It is possible for sperm, upon entering the urethra, to go back into the bladder rather than forward into the penis. This is called *retrograde ejaculation*. Retrograde ejaculation may be a result of the effect of certain drugs or medications such as tranquilizers or antihypertensive medication. It may be a product of nerve degeneration or in rare cases may follow a prostatectomy. The diagnosis can be made if no sperm are emitted from the penis but there are sperm in a urine sample obtained immediately following a dry ejaculation.

When retrograde ejaculation is a result of medication, the doctor can treat it by changing drugs or diminishing drug dose. When it is the result of other problems, the patient may be treated by being catheterized after ejaculation. Then the doctor can obtain the sperm deposited within the bladder and use this for artificial insemination.

If the penis has the hole that is usually at its tip in an abnormal position, delivery of sperm within the vagina becomes very dif-

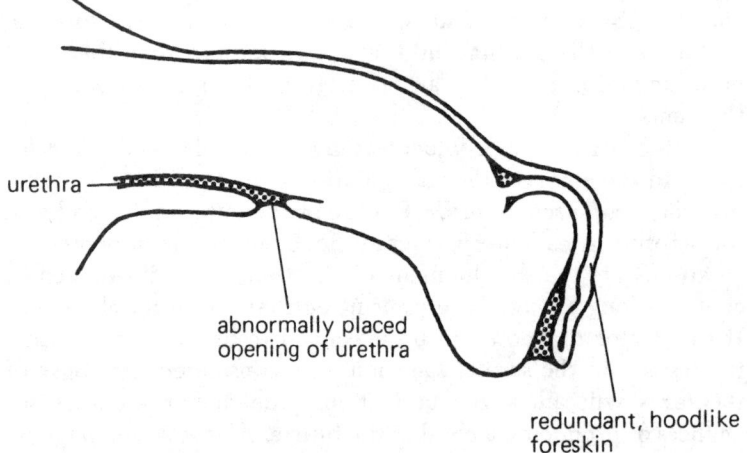

urethra

abnormally placed
opening of urethra

redundant, hoodlike
foreskin

Figure 4.2 *The opening of the urethra, the tube which carries urine and sperm, is in an abnormal position, away from the end of the penis on its underside. Because of its location, the normal placement of sperm within the vagina may be prevented.*

ficult. *Hypospadias,* a condition where the opening of the penis is on the underside, back from the tip, is one of the more common forms of this abnormality. Instead of sperm being deposited within the vagina, next to the cervix, within the cervical mucus, it may be deposited in the outer third of the vagina so that not enough, if any, will ever reach the cervix. Therapy for this is simply to have the man masturbate to obtain a specimen of sperm and deliver it to the woman by artificial insemination. Since the sperm should be normal in every other respect, the probability of achieving success should be quite good. (See Figure 4.2.)

Infection

Infection may also cause male infertility. Any process causing inflammation of the testes may significantly damage the cells producing sperm. An inflammation of the testes is referred to as *orchitis*. When men contract mumps after puberty, approximately 25 percent have damage to the testicles that later results in reproductive problems. When a man develops an orchitis the testes become swollen and very painful to the touch. If a piece of tissue is removed from the testis at a later date, microscopic examination shows definite damage to some of the sperm-producing elements and atrophy of the testis itself. This damage is irreversible. Gonorrhea may also produce damage to the sperm-producing elements of the testes. Gonorrhea should be treated promptly not only to prevent its spread but also to maintain fertility.

Another infectious agent, one between a virus and a bacterium in structure, is *chlamydia*. In men this organism is frequently the cause of "nonspecific" urethritis. Nonspecific urethritis is a term used to identify a cluster of symptoms most frequently including burning on urination, urinary frequency, and a discharge from the end of the penis when the usual cultures for gonorrhea and other bacterial organisms are negative. More recently, sophisticated culture techniques have shown the presence of chlamydia in such cases. With the growing awareness of chlamydia and more extensive screening techniques, it has been found that chlamydia is the leading cause of sexually transmitted infections in the United States, surpassing even gonorrhea.

Chlamydia can produce symptoms similar to those of a urinary tract infection or even gonorrhea. Chlamydia usually does not directly affect sperm production but can produce scarring and potential obstruction of the epididymis, which is part of the pathway used to carry sperm from the testes to the penis. The organism is usually sensitive to tetracycline or erythromycin. Early treatment can prevent epididymal scarring and resulting obstruction, so chlamydial infections in men are not a major cause of male infertility. The main concern is that chlamydial infections may produce few if any complaints. Thus, chlamydial infection with no symptoms can be passed back and forth between the two members of a couple. In the woman, a chlamydial infection may be totally without symptoms. The result is that this organism can produce extensive damage to the Fallopian tubes resulting in infertility without ever producing any warning. Without early warning, successful treatment may be impossible.

Another infectious agent similar to chlamydia, also between a virus and a bacterium in structure, is *mycoplasma*. Genital mycoplasmas can be divided into two subgroups: *U. urealyticum* and *mycoplasma hominis*. One particular subgroup of mycoplasma is frequently discussed as an infectious agent leading to infertility. This subgroup is called a T-strain mycoplasma (or T-mycoplasma for short), and is now referred to as U. urealyticum. Both groups, U. urealyticum and M. hominis, have been statistically associated with infertility though their precise role is still a product of much debate. Nevertheless, in at least some cases, ureaplasma seems to fasten itself to sperm cells and render them less mobile and less capable of producing fertilization. The diagnosis of mycoplasma infection is very difficult to make. The ideal way is to take a sample of semen, culture it, and let the organism grow. However, ureaplasma does not seem to cooperate and does not always grow well in a laboratory culture medium. Furthermore, mycoplasma has been found in people with no reproductive problems. In years to come, we hope to see its role in infertility clarified.

Genetic Causes

There are also genetic reasons for the inability of a man to cause conception. Normal males have forty-six chromosomes with an X and a Y chromosome, referred to as 46 XY. Normal females have forty-six chromosomes with two X chromosomes, referred to as 46 XX. An abnormal chromosomal composition frequently compromises reproductive ability. If instead of having XY sex chromosomes, a man has two X chromosomes along with the Y—an XXY chromosomal pattern—*he* would most probably not be able to reproduce. A man with an XXY pattern has slightly widened hips and slightly longer than normal extremities. His breasts may be minimally enlarged and his testes small. A semen analysis will fail to show any sperm present and a biopsy of his testes will show no sperm. An XXY male is known as having *Klinefelter's syndrome.* In some rare cases a man with Klinefelter's syndrome can produce sperm but in numbers so small as to make producing pregnancy virtually impossible. Even though a man with this syndrome has an extra X chromosome, in areas other than reproduction he is a normal man and should not fear that he is a cross between a man and a woman.

Hormonal Causes

The *hormonal* causes of infertility in men include the malfunctioning of almost any of the glands of the endocrine system. The pituitary gland can cause infertility because of one of two kinds of deficiencies. The man may have a selective deficiency of FSH and LH. These hormones are necessary for the development of sperm cells and for the production of *testosterone,* the hormone responsible for male secondary sex characteristics. If the pituitary gland produces all other hormones except FSH and LH it is said to have a selective deficiency of these hormones. One such clinical state is described as *Kallman's syndrome* and is usually associated with defects in the sense of smell and occasionally in deformities of the face. Another possibility is that the pituitary gland may fail to produce almost all of its hormones, not just FSH and LH, resulting in poorly or nonfunctioning testes, thyroid gland, and adrenal gland. This is called *panhypopituitarism.*

A doctor can diagnose selective FSH and LH deficiency or a panhypopituitarism by drawing and testing blood for levels of the pituitary hormones. Deficiencies of just FSH and LH indicate a selective deficiency whereas total absence of all pituitary hormones points to a panhypopituitarism problem. In the latter case physical examination shows signs consistent with thyroid and adrenal problems. There may also be poor functioning of the thyroid or the adrenal gland unrelated to any pituitary problems.

The signs and symptoms are often so subtle or even nonexistent that physical examination is of little help. That is why the lab studies are important.

Underfunctioning of thyroid or adrenal glands can be discovered by studying the blood levels of thyroxine in the first case and cortisol in the second. Occasionally defects in the entire chemistry of the adrenal gland may exist. These can be determined by examining all the urine collected in a twenty-four–hour period for biochemical products of the adrenal gland. Tests are usually done for substances known as 17-hydroxycorticosteroids, 17-ketosteroids and pregnantriol.

Drug and Medication Use

Both cocaine and heavy marijuana use have been associated with a decrease in the number of sperm cells being produced and a reduction in the quality of these cells. The result is that both these drugs reduce male fertility. It is difficult to say what the smallest amount of a drug is that a man can use without affecting his fertility. A man who has a high normal sperm count may be able to get away with the use of some recreational drugs. Though his count may drop, at times by 50 percent or more, it may still remain within the normal range. Another individual having a low normal count, using exactly the same amount of recreational drugs, may find that his count will go well below normal and he will be essentially infertile. The best rule is to refrain from using any recreational drugs. Alcohol and nicotine may also be considered recreational drugs, and a man who has a borderline sperm sample should restrict his use of them.

Environment

Environment plays a role in the cause of infertility. Radiation will affect any rapidly dividing cell population. Since the cells producing sperm belong to this class, these cells may be quite sensitive to radiation damage. Following significant radiation it may take up to two years for the return of sperm cell production. If sperm cell production has not returned four years after radiation it probably will never return. Heat applied locally around the testes can also affect sperm cell production. Men who spend most of their time sitting at the job, such as truck drivers, taxi drivers, and office desk workers, tend to have a lower sperm count than the general population.

Over the last several years there has been much discussion over whether or not the quality of sperm production throughout the world has deteriorated. Specialists in male infertility are markedly divided in the assessment of published findings. Several publications seem to show that in the last twenty years, the number of sperm cells produced and the percentage of normally moving sperm cells have each diminished in the general male population. If this finding is real, it may represent the effects of pollution in our environment and the increase of recreational drug use. More men are surviving after chemotherapy for cancer and more drugs are used to treat diseases which in the past were not treatable. The result is that more men are exposed to substances that can potentially affect sperm quality and numbers. There is disagreement about whether the apparent decline in quality is real, and, if it has any clinical significance.

The catalog of agents that can interfere with sperm production is large. A partial list includes: alcohol, tobacco smoke, marijuana smoke, certain antibiotics, lead, X-rays, plutonium, DDT, polychlorinated biphenyls (PCBs), hetachloral phenal, DBCP, kepone, and dioxyn. One ingredient of agent orange that contains dioxyn was sprayed for years on power lines and rights of way in the United States.

Drugs typically used to treat many stress-related illnesses also have effects on sperm production. Tagamet (cimetidine), used to treat ulcers, and Azulfidine (sulphasalazine), used to treat ulcerative colitis, each are capable of reducing sperm counts. I am not questioning the medical appropriateness of using these drugs. We live in a society where there is an increased need for such medication, but we must be conscious of the ramifications of their use.

We cannot go back to a simpler life, but as a society we must be more aware of what we are putting into our bodies. Perhaps we should ask ourselves more frequently, "Is this drug really

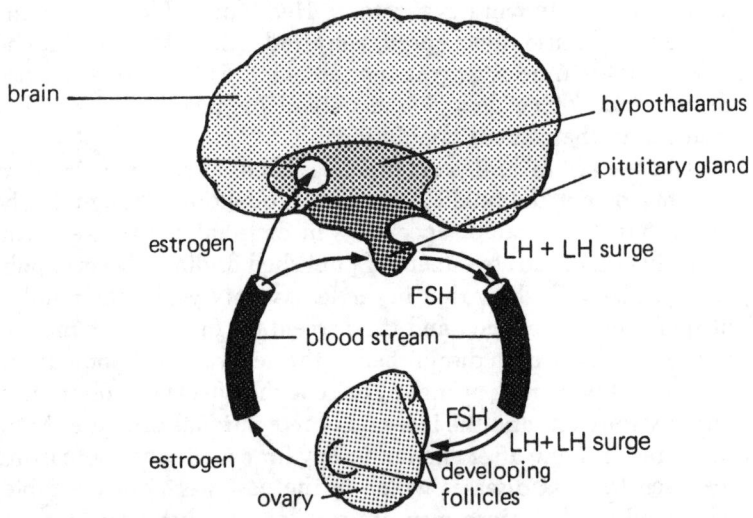

Figure 4.3 *Normal hypothalamus, pituitary gland, and ovary interacting.*

needed?" or "Is there another way of treating this problem?" If the answer is clearly that the drug is the best choice, then we have made an educated decision. If there is another way of accomplishing the desired end, perhaps that should be taken.

EVALUATING THE WOMAN

Anovulation

Female factor infertility has several causes, the most common being a failure to ovulate. This is called *anovulation*, literally nonovulation. Anovulation can occur because the ovary has exhausted its supply of eggs and is no longer functioning. This is called *ovarian failure* and usually occurs in menopausal women in their mid-forties. When this occurs in a woman of twenty or thirty, it is called *premature ovarian failure*. Fortunately, unless

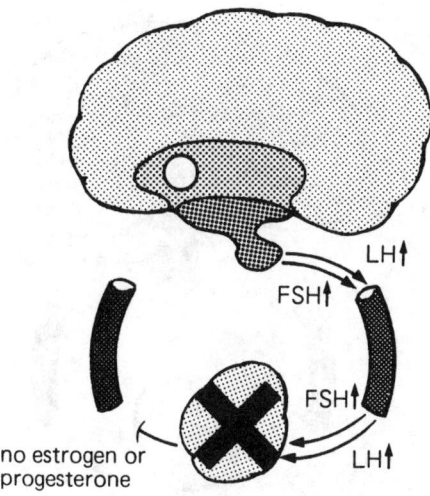

Figure 4.4 *Ovarian failure. The ovary fails to respond to FSH and LH stimulation. No estrogen or progesterone is produced. No ovulation occurs. Blood levels of FSH and LH are high. Blood studies: FSH and LH are high; estrogen is almost absent.*

the woman has had abdominal radiotherapy or surgical damage to both ovaries, premature ovarian failure is an uncommon cause of infertility. I say "fortunately" because there is no treatment at this time for documented premature ovarian failure. In order to confirm the fact that a woman has exhausted her supply of eggs, many physicians will take an ovarian biopsy (surgically cutting a small section of the ovary) to confirm the diagnosis under the microscope. Hormonal studies, FSH and LH levels also may be used. (See Figures 4.3 and 4.4.)

It is more common for the ovary to be functioning but for there to be insufficient hormonal stimulus to cause ovulation. FSH and LH are produced by the pituitary gland under the influence of the hypothalamus. A certain baseline amount of these hormones must be produced to stimulate and ready the ovary to ovulate. Then, at midcycle, with the specific stimulation of the

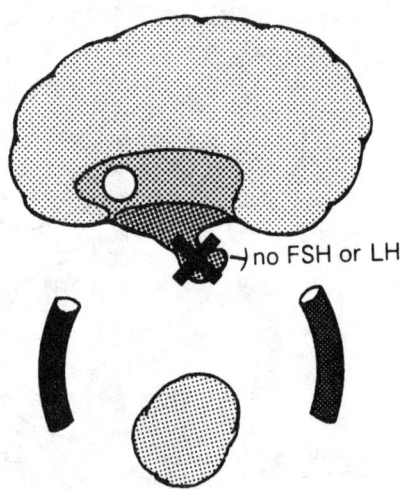

Figure 4.5 *Pituitary problem. No FSH and LH are produced. Therefore the ovary receives no stimulation. Thus, no estrogen or progesterone is made and no ovulation occurs. Blood studies: FSH and LH are almost absent; estrogen is almost absent.*

hypothalamus, the pituitary releases a massive amount of FSH and LH, producing a sudden surge of these substances within the bloodstream. It is this surge of LH and FSH that produces ovulation. The baseline levels of FSH and LH ready the ovary for ovulation and cause it to produce its normal levels of estrogen. Following ovulation, these lower levels help to maintain the corpus luteum and allow the ovary to produce estrogen and progesterone.

If the pituitary is unable to produce FSH and LH because of damage to the cells that make these hormones, then the ovary is not stimulated to become ready for ovulation. The result is essentially no FSH and LH in your blood, little or no estrogen produced from your ovary, and no ovulation. The pituitary problem is causing the lack of ovulation. (See Figure 4.5.)

If you have a functioning ovary and pituitary but a hypothal-

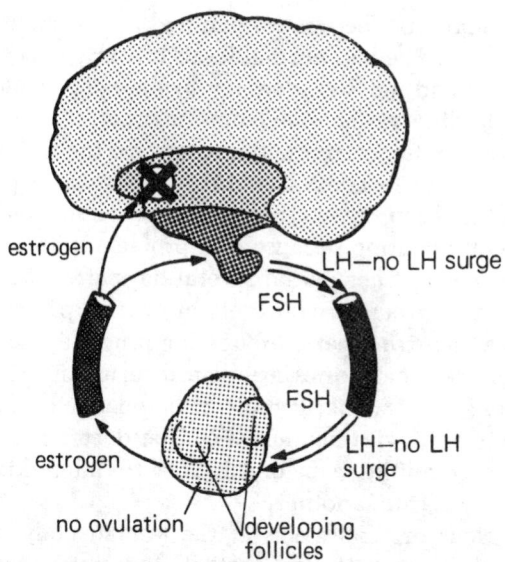

Figure 4.6 *Hypothalamic problem. FSH and LH are being produced, but no LH surge occurs. Since the LH surge is necessary for ovulation, no ovulation occurs. Blood studies: FSH and LH are of normal range; estrogen is of normal range; progesterone is absent.*

amus that does not stimulate ovulation, the result would be FSH and LH produced in the usual baseline manner and estrogen produced from the ovary. No midcycle surge of the pituitary hormones would occur and there would be no ovulation. A blood sample in this case would show normal levels of LH and FSH and normal levels of estrogen. Here a malfunctioning hypothalamus causes nonovulation. (See Figure 4.6.)

I have just described three cases of failure to ovulate. The first was a woman with premature ovarian failure. Her ovaries have exhausted their supply of eggs. She has a very high level of FSH and LH in her blood, low levels of estrogen, and no ovulation. The second woman had a problem with her pituitary resulting in extremely low levels of FSH, LH, and estrogen in her blood and no ovulation. The last woman had a malfunctioning of her hypothalamus. She had normal levels of FSH, LH, and estrogen in her blood and she, too, does not ovulate. Their blood samples will help to differentiate one from the other.

Another way to determine the reason for the lack of ovulation is for the doctor to administer progesterone or a progesterone-like drug. If the problem is hypothalamic anovulation, that is, if she is not ovulating because of a problem with her hypothalamus, she will get her period several days after she receives the progesterone. If there are pituitary or ovarian problems, she will not have a menstrual period following progesterone.

Though these categories are described as distinct groups for the purpose of this book, it must be emphasized that in real life they may merge with one another. The doctor may have to do tests well beyond the scope of this book to differentiate one kind of anovulation from another.

The various organ systems of the human body interact and remain in balance with one another. It is not uncommon for a problem in one system to be reflected by an improper functioning of another organ system. This is the case with hypothalamic anovulation. Not infrequently, hypothalamic anovulation may be a result of a glandular problem unassociated with the female reproductive system. Hypothalamic anovulation may be the first sign of an overfunctioning or underfunctioning of the thyroid or adrenal gland or of an early diabetic state.

With hypothalamic anovulation a woman need not cease ovulating altogether but may manage to ovulate two, three, or even four times a year. Though this is better than producing no eggs at all, it is still not very much help if she is seeking a pregnancy. Rather than having twelve opportunities for pregnancy in a year, there may be only two, three, or four. With regular ovulation, the time that a woman is fertile can be predicted month after month. When a woman ovulates irregularly, she generally does not know precisely when she is fertile, and the chances of having sexual relations at that time may be pure luck. So whether hypothalamic anovulation results in a total absence of the release of eggs or in an infrequent, irregular ovulation, it should be treated.

Other Hormonal Problems

Hormonal causes *that do not* interfere with ovulation may also result in infertility in women. In some cases the patient may have either an over- or underactivity of the thyroid or adrenal gland. One cause may be diabetes. In some cases this may affect ovulation, but in other cases the abnormal functioning may be so slight that ovulation occurs but pregnancy may not. It is not always obvious why this should happen. It may be that the woman becomes pregnant but then loses the pregnancy so quickly that she never misses her period. The pregnancy test never turns positive and she is never aware that she had become pregnant in the first place. Or a woman may become pregnant but, because of hormonal problems, lose the pregnancy several weeks after conception.

Progesterone, the hormone produced by the ovary after ovulation, is necessary for the survival of the newly fertilized egg. It works by acting upon the lining of the uterus, the endometrium, to convert it into a tissue capable of nourishing the fertilized egg. This nourishing tissue, called secretory endometrium, constantly changes in structure following ovulation. The change in microscopic structure must take place in a certain sequence and at a certain rate over approximately fourteen days. The sequence of changes is produced by progesterone and is dependent upon the amount and rate of this hormone's release. If progesterone is produced for too short a period of time or in too small a quantity, the required changes in the endometrium may occur too slowly or not at all. The result is that the fertilized egg may not be able to survive in the uterine cavity. This is frequently called an *inadequate luteal phase* or a *luteal phase defect*. Such a progesterone deficiency may be a cause of infertility in apparently normally ovulating woman. A doctor can evaluate blood levels of progesterone by drawing a sample of blood approximately one week after ovulation. A more precise assessment of the second half of the cycle, and thereby progesterone effect, can be done by sampling the tissue lining of the uterus to see if the appropriate progesterone changes have occurred. This procedure is called an *endometrial biopsy*. Some investigators feel that progesterone deficiencies are associated not only with infertility but also with miscarriages in early pregnancy. Sometimes these two problems may masquerade as one another. If a woman becomes pregnant but loses the embryo so early that she bleeds at the time of her expected period, then the pregnancy loss will appear to be infertility. If the environment within the uterine cavity is very much out of phase in development, then the fertilized egg will never be able to implant in the lining of the uterus. Here, even though a couple may be producing embryos on a regular basis, infertility will still result. Thus early loss of pregnancy can merge with infertility and both can be intimately associated with progesterone deficiencies.

Determining whether or not a hormonal deficiency exists is relatively simple. The doctor studies blood and, in some cases, urine samples for the hormonal products of the gland being investigated. The doctor can screen for diabetes by studying the blood sugar level. If the blood sugar level is abnormal, more detailed studies of sugar metabolism can be done with a glucose tolerance test.

Structural Problems

The third major category of causes of infertility in women is that of *structural abnormalities*. It is obvious that if a woman does not have a uterus, or Fallopian tubes, or a vagina, pregnancy, by ordinary means, is impossible. Inflammation involving the Fallopian tubes as a result of gonorrhea or acute appendicitis, may scar the tissue around the Fallopian tubes, possibly within the walls of the tubes, preventing their function, and partially obstructing the channel within the tube. In order for the Fallopian tube to function it must have the delicate, folded lining within a muscular tube that is capable of free movement. The tube must be capable of a coordinated contraction, moving the sperm in one direction, the egg in the other direction, and the fertilized egg back toward the uterus. If an infection has caused scarring of the Fallopian tube, the delicate lining of the structure may have been irreversibly damaged. Muscle fibers

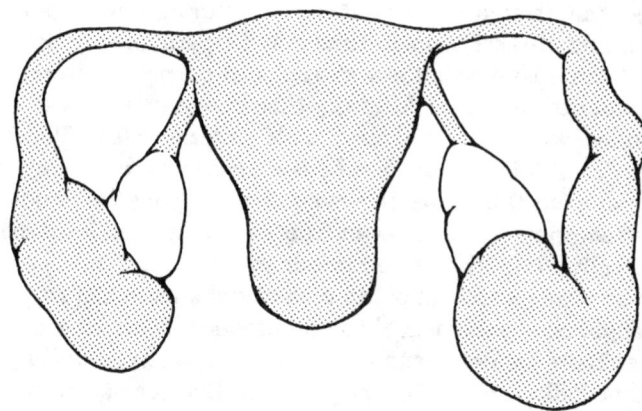

Figure 4.7 *Hydrosalpinx. Both tubes are closed and enlarged into two thin-walled, saclike structures. These tubes are unable to pick up an egg.*

within the wall may have been destroyed and replaced by fibrous scar tissue. This scar tissue is not capable of contracting and will upset the coordinated movement of the tube. The channel within the tube itself may develop scar tissue, which will grow and close off the tube.

The end of the Fallopian tube is a funnel-shaped, freely movable, highly specialized structure called the *fimbria*. It is designed to pick up the egg when it is released from the ovary. Its ability to move freely is an important factor in catching the egg. When the fimbria becomes inflamed, whether as a result of infection or irritation, the delicate folds may stick together. Instead of the end of the tube being open and funnel shaped, it may be drawn together like the end of a laundry bag with its strings pulled tightly. In severe cases, the opening may be totally obliterated and the end of the tube may appear club shaped. (See Figure 4.7.) When the end of the tube is completely obstructed, as a result of an infection such as gonorrhea, the entire Fallopian tube fills with pus and turns into a large sac. With time, the infection is gone but the sac with its scarring remains. The lining of the Fallopian tube may be permanently destroyed and the muscle within the wall replaced partially or completely with connective tissue. After the tube has healed, instead of being filled with pus, it is filled with a sterile, clear fluid. This scarred, fluid-filled, saclike tube is a nonfunctioning remnant of the Fallopian tube. The only way of remedying this problem is by attempting surgical reconstruction. This will be discussed more fully in the chapter on treatment.

In an attempt to wall off an area of irritation when an area of the abdomen is inflamed, the body produces layers of connective tissue. These bands of connective tissue, known as *adhesions*, may hold the Fallopian tube in such a position that egg pickup becomes almost impossible and infertility results. (See Figure 4.8.)

Gonorrhea or pelvic infection is not the only cause of adhesions around the tubes and ovaries. Any irritation will result in inflammation, which in some cases is followed by adhesion formation. Some women are much more susceptible to adhesion formation than others.

Today, chlamydia, an organism appearing to be somewhat like a virus and a bacterium, is the leading cause of reproductive infections in the United States. Chlamydia is capable of causing a silent, insidious pelvic infection that can produce significant Fallopian tube damage and extensive pelvic irritation. Because the infections frequently produce slight symptoms or none at all, they may result in significant destruction before any treatment is begun. Sometimes no treatment is provided because the infection may run its course without resulting in any complaints whatsoever.

Both chlamydia and mycoplasma are fastidious organisms, meaning they are difficult to culture. When we take a swab of tissue thought to be infected with either one of these organisms and place it in culture medium, an environment designed to make the organisms grow, the organisms may still fail to multiply. A negative culture for chlamydia and/or mycoplasma does not mean the organism is not present. Thus, one of the classic and basic studies to demonstrate the presence or absence of a microorganism may not be valid for these two infectious agents.

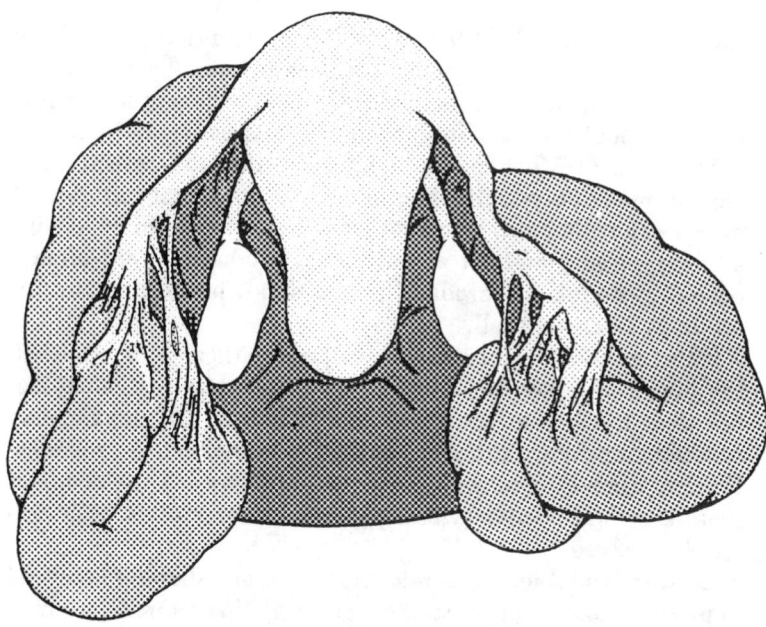

Figure 4.8 *Adhesions immobilizing the tube. Connective tissue bands (adhesions) may form around the Fallopian tubes preventing the fimbria from picking up an ovum or actually obstructing the tube.*

To get around this difficulty, other studies have been designed to prove the existence of these organisms. We can use special stains for chlamydia to help locate the organism on a slide. We can test slides or swabs thought to contain chlamydia for special enzymes present in the organisms. Unfortunately, at times these studies also fail to pick up the presence of the infectious agent.

Another way of screening for chlamydia and mycoplasma is to look for antibodies to these organisms. Whenever someone has been infected, the body produces a very specific and unique substance to attack the invader. This substance is called an *antibody* and should be unique to the particular agent. If a person is infected by organism A, the body will produce antibodies to A. By testing someone's blood for antibodies to A, a doctor should be able to tell whether or not he has been infected by that agent. However, long after the infection, the body will continue to produce antibodies to that organism. Thus, finding antibodies to organism A does not tell the doctor whether the patient has a current infection or antibodies left over from a past infection. A doctor can distinguish a current from a past infection by looking at the type and amount of antibodies produced. Very often a current infection will produce high antibody levels; later on, the antibody levels will fall.

Thus, antibody testing is not foolproof either. It does not tell the doctor whether the infection is a current or past infection, nor does it tell the location of the infection. Chlamydia may produce respiratory problems as well as reproductive problems. Finding antibodies in the bloodstream will not tell the doctor if there is a reproductive system problem or some other body system is involved.

Cultures and smears can miss organisms and therefore are said to produce false negative studies, meaning that an infection may be present but might have been missed by the laboratory test. Antibody studies usually do not miss active infections, but they may give positive readings long after the infection is gone. These tests are said to produce "false positive" studies: there will be a positive result even when an infection is not present at the time of testing. We tend to use antibody studies as well as cultures when testing for chlamydia.

If a fluid-filled ovarian cyst forms and breaks, the liquid that comes out may irritate the tissue covering the tubes and an adhesion may form. If the ovary bleeds excessively from an area where an egg was released, adhesions may follow. Using an intrauterine contraceptive, an IUD, can cause tubal adhesions to form in some women. In experimental animals, a high fever can cause a general reaction throughout the body that is sometimes followed by pelvic adhesions. The same thing may occur in humans. This may be important since almost every adult has had a high fever at some time during childhood. It is then not surprising that a particular woman has tubal adhesions but rather that not every woman has them.

Endometriosis is another cause of tubal scarring. The lining of the uterus, the endometrium, is composed of actively growing tissue that expands during a woman's menstrual cycle and crumbles around the time of her period. For unknown reasons, some women have this tissue outside the uterus. When this occurs it is called endometriosis. The ovaries, the outer surface of the Fallopian tubes, and the uterosacral ligaments on the back of the uterus are the most common locations for this misplaced endometrium. When these areas of endometriosis expand during the cycle they become very sensitive to the touch. If, during sexual activities, these areas are shaken or touched, they usually produce significant pain. The result is painful sexual relations or *dyspareunia*. (See Figure 4.9.)

During menstruation the areas of endometriosis may crumble and produce a pasty material that is extremely irritating to the surrounding tissues. This results in severe pain, called *dysmenorrhea*, during menstruation. This irritating material may actually destroy some of the tissue around it. As the area heals, fibrous connective tissue replaces the damaged tissue and a scar forms. The area around this becomes inflamed and later adhesions form. The end product is a Fallopian tube with areas of muscle destroyed and scarred, held in an abnormal position by adhesions.

There are many degrees of endometriosis. In some cases there may be areas with little scarring and no adhesions that are so small that they would escape observation by all but the most diligent physician. In other cases the areas may produce masses that are so large they fill the entire lower abdomen. Infertility may result in women with even the smallest areas of endometriosis well away from the tubes and ovaries.

Endometriosis is usually treatable by medication and/or surgery. This will be discussed in Chapter 9.

Connective tissue may form over the surface of the ovary. In a healed state, that is, after an inflammation has subsided, the connective tissue remains. This connective tissue actively prevents the egg from escaping from the surface of the ovary, thus preventing its pickup by the fimbria of the Fallopian tube. The only way of correcting this is by surgically removing the connective tissue. This too will be discussed in Chapters 6 and 12.

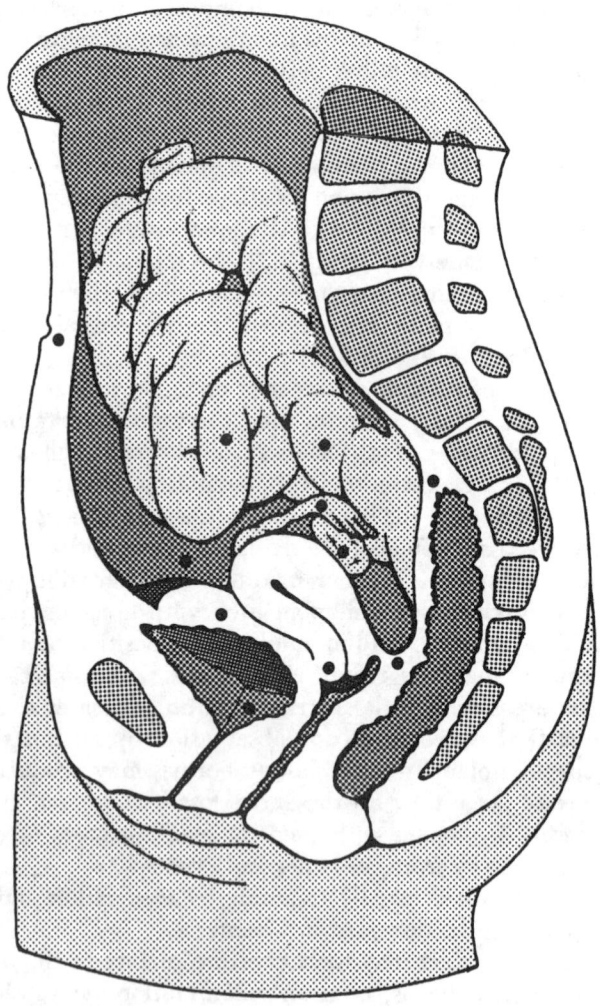

Figure 4.9 *Endometriosis. Some of the possible sites of endometriosis are shown.*

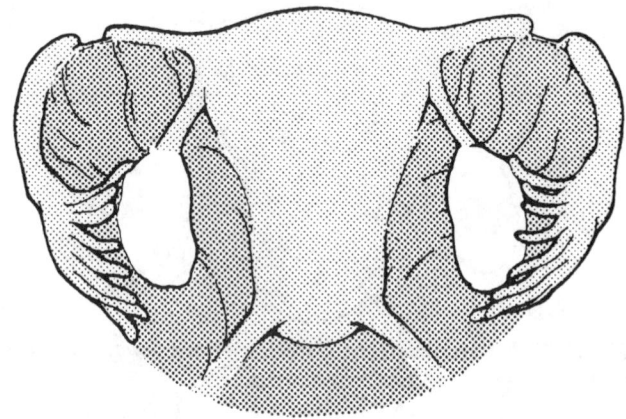

Figure 4.10 *Tubal ligation (sterilization). Small segments of the middle of the tubes have been removed.*

Infertility may be the result of sterilization. A tubal ligation may have been done where a segment of the Fallopian tube has been removed and the two free ends of the tube healed closed. The result is a double obstruction within the channel of the Fallopian tube preventing the movement of the egg and the sperm so that they may not reach one another. If the woman now desires pregnancy the only way of remedying this situation is by surgically reconnecting the tubes. It is also possible that in an attempt to produce permanent sterilization, the surgeon removed the entire Fallopian tube or the segment containing the fimbria. If this is the case, with the available surgical techniques at this time, there is no way of replacing or reconstructing such a tube and restoring fertility. The only way of achieving a pregnancy without Fallopian tubes is by *in vitro fertilization.* (See Figures 4.10, 4.11, 4.12.) (See Chapter 11.)

There are various kinds of surgical sterilization available today. In the chapter on therapy I discuss the potential for reversing these surgical procedures.

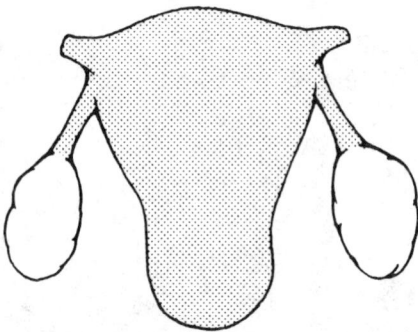

Figure 4.11 *Tubal sterilization. Here the entire tubes have been removed. This is known as a salpingectomy.*

Infertility may also be the result of an abnormality in the structure of the uterine cavity. This may be a wall (or *septum*) extending down into the cavity or it may be the deformity of the cavity by a benign tumor called a leiomyoma or, in more conventional language, a *fibroid*. Occasionally, the front and back walls of the uterine cavity may become stuck together. This may be the result of an infection or scarring of the uterine cavity. The

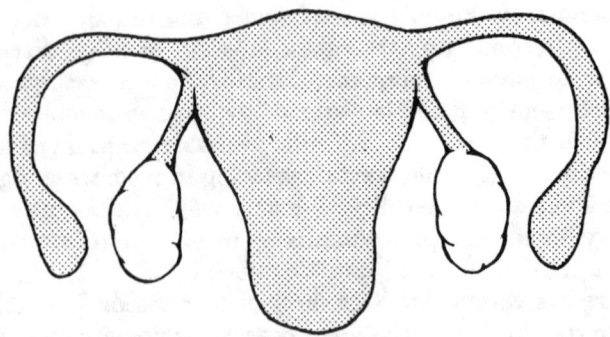

Figure 4.12 *Tubal sterilization. Here the fimbria have been removed from both tubes. This is known as a fimbriectomy.*

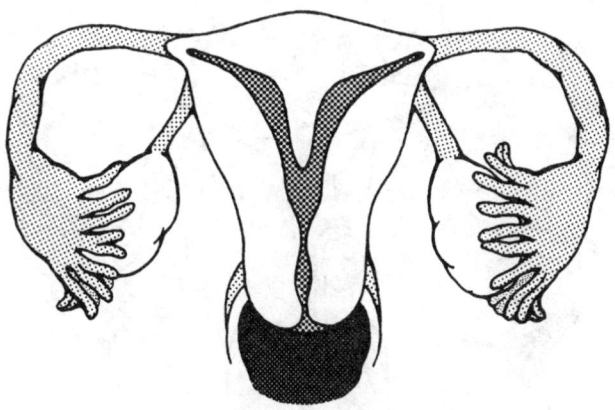

Figure 4.13 *Uterus with a septum.*

front and back walls of the cavity adhere to each other through the formation of scar tissue very much like the scar tissue previously discussed which may form around the Fallopian tubes. The presence of this scar tissue, which obliterates the cavity, is referred to as *Asherman's syndrome*. (See Figures 4.13 and 4.14.)

A doctor can discover an abnormality of the uterine cavity by using a *hysterosalpingogram*, that is, an X-ray of the uterine cavity, or by placing a specialized telescope called a *hysteroscope* in the uterine cavity through the cervix and visually examining the contents of the cavity.

Abnormalities of the uterine cavity other than Asherman's syndrome usually do not prevent pregnancy, but hinder the development of a pregnancy, causing spontaneous abortion (miscarriage). When a patient has a history of repeated pregnancy loss, the doctor should consider the possibility of an intrauterine abnormality.

The fourth kind of structural abnormality that may exist in the female reproductive tract is something called an *incompetent cervix*. The opening to the uterus, which is found at the innermost part of the vagina, is called the cervix. It has circular mus-

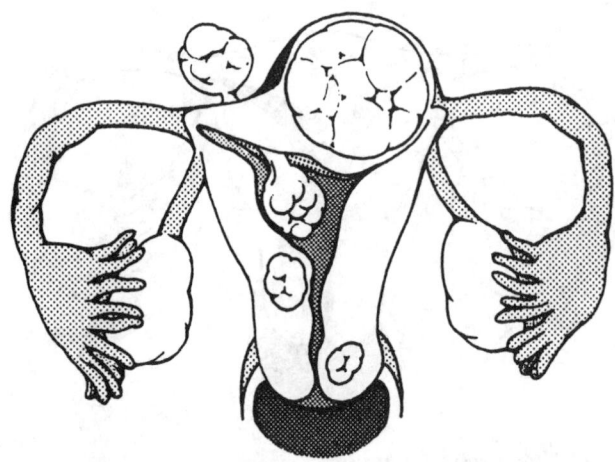

Figure 4.14 *Fibroids. These noncancerous tumors distort the surface of the uterus or may actually compress and close off the Fallopian tubes. In this way they may result in infertility or miscarriage.*

cle and connective tissue running up into the body of the uterus and around the opening of the uterus, very much like the drawstrings on a laundry bag. Once a woman conceives, the pregnancy grows within the uterus. When the woman stands up in the ordinary, everyday walking position, the weight of the pregnancy is exerted downward against the cervix. It is the job of this connective tissue to keep the opening of the cervix closed until the time for labor. If these fibers do not do their job, the cervix will gradually open as the weight of the growing pregnancy is exerted against it until, sometime in mid-pregnancy, the patient will suddenly feel a splash or gush of some fluid and the fetus will be passed painlessly. This is unlike other kinds of miscarriage where a woman feels cramps and discomfort very much like real labor. Miscarriages associated with an incompetent cervix are most commonly painless.

When the Cervix Does Not Work Properly

Improper functioning of the cervix also causes infertility. In order for sperm to enter the uterine cavity and the Fallopian tube to fertilize the egg, they must swim through a large quantity of watery mucus secreted by the cervix. This mucus acts as a medium through which the sperm may swim to reach the uterine cavity and the Fallopian tube. Some women produce too little cervical mucus. Others produce cervical mucus that is so thick that sperm cannot penetrate it. In either case, the cervical mucus acts as a barrier rather than as a means through which the sperm may reach the uterine cavity and the egg. A doctor can diagnose this fairly simply by doing a *postcoital test,* sometimes called a *Simms-Huhner test,* at the time of ovulation. It is at this time that the cervical mucus should be present in its greatest volume and in its most favorable quality to support the life of the sperm. If only a small quantity is found or if the texture of the mucus is thick rather than watery, the diagnosis of poor quality cervical mucus is made. As discussed in Chapter 6, this is easily treatable.

MALE–FEMALE INTERACTION

In order for pregnancy to be established, a man and woman must have sexual relations at least once or, ideally, several times around the time of ovulation for several cycles in succession. A couple should not begin to be concerned until they have had intercourse regularly for one year without the production of a pregnancy. If a couple has relations less frequently or has intercourse at the wrong time of the cycle, pregnancy cannot occur. The only way to determine whether or not the problem is one of poor timing is for the doctor to take a very careful history at the first visit. For this reason it is very helpful if both the man and woman are present at the first visit to the doctor's office for an infertility evaluation. The history obtained will review the frequency, the technique, and the timing of sexual relations.

There may also be certain social and cultural problems. For example, Orthodox Jews cannot have relations for one week after the cessation of a woman's menstrual flow. If the woman ovulates on cycle day fourteen and her period goes past cycle day eight, then intercourse will never occur at the time of ovulation and pregnancy cannot occur. Such factors must be taken into account in evaluating the problems of an infertile couple.

Another problem in male–female interaction is the actual mechanics of having intercourse. It is possible that the man is unable to obtain sufficient rigidity of his penis to penetrate the woman's vagina. It is also possible that the muscle tone and the tension of the woman is such that she constricts her vagina and its penetration by a normal penis is impossible. In either event, the result is that the man cannot deposit his sperm in the woman's vagina. Occasionally, when vaginal tone is maintained to such a degree that vaginal entrance is impossible, called *vaginismus*, the man may place his penis within the woman's urethral opening. The urethra is the tube which drains the bladder and so is the opening through which urine flows when a woman urinates. If this opening is the area of least resistance, then it is possible to have urethral intercourse instead of vaginal intercourse. This is extremely unusual, but nevertheless the doctor must consider it. Similarly, it is possible to have rectal intercourse when entrance into the vagina cannot be accomplished. Some couples may have had regular rectal intercourse without realizing it. When a man with good semen specimens and his partner are asked to have intercourse so a postcoital test can be done and there are no sperm in the vagina, then a problem of sexual technique seems very likely. The remedy frequently involves further education, investigation of sexual techniques, and occasionally sex therapy. The results of this type of treatment are excellent.

Another problem is that of antibodies. If a man and a woman are having intercourse properly and nonmoving sperm cells are found within the cervical mucus, the doctor must consider if there is something within the cervical mucus or within the man's seminal fluid that is killing the sperm. One possible explanation is that the body's defense system, known as its *immunological system*, may be attacking the sperm and killing it.

The human body has a very special defense system. It can

recognize which cells belong to it and which cells belong to something or somebody else. Any cells that are foreign, that is, that do not belong to that particular individual, are recognized as potential invaders and are attacked. This works out rather well if the cell that is attacked is a disease-causing microorganism. The cells are attacked by covering them with a thin layer of antibodies made by the body, known as *gamma globulin.*

This renders the cells inactive and prepares them for destruction by other specialized cells of the body. Occasionally this defense system makes an error. Cells that are part of that individual's body mistakenly may be identified as foreign and may be attacked. The result is a partial breakdown of the organ system to which the attacked cells belong. If the attacked cells are part of the surface of a joint, then the patient may develop arthritis. If the cells being attacked belong to the lungs, then the patient develops asthma.

Occasionally, though rarely, a man may become sensitive or allergic to his own sperm cells. In this case, he would produce sperm in normal numbers that may or may not move around when examined under the microscope, but are unable to fertilize an egg because they are coated with gamma globulin. In another case a woman may produce antibodies to sperm cells. These antibodies may be in the blood, cervical mucus, or in the secretions within the uterine cavity. When normal sperm interacts with the secretions containing antibodies the sperm cells are covered with gamma globulin and rendered inactive.

The postcoital tests in such cases may show reduced or total absence of movement of the sperm cells. It is also possible that though each sperm cell is covered with gamma globulin, its movement is not reduced, only its ability to fertilize an egg. The postcoital test would then be normal but fertilization would still be impossible. Fortunately, this paradoxical situation is extremely unusual. Thus, if a postcoital test is normal and all other studies fail to show a cause for a couple's infertility, immunological studies to reveal antisperm antibodies in the man or woman are still indicated.

In a certain sense, the immunological system mistakenly may create a toxic environment for the sperm cell, making it impossible for the sperm to fertilize an egg. Some investigators feel that other things may cause a toxic environment. In some cases the environment can be so bad as to actually kill the sperm cells. A microorganism identified as mycoplasma has been incriminated as a possible culprit. This microorganism has been found in the cervical mucus and the seminal fluid of couples with unexplained infertility or recurrent miscarriage. Unfortunately, the microorganism also has been found in couples with normal reproductive histories. Nevertheless when some couples are given antibiotic therapy and the organisms are eradicated, fertility returns. To make the diagnosis, the doctor takes cervical mucus from the woman and seminal fluid from the man and adds it to a culture medium that will allow the microorganism to grow. If the organism appears on culture, antibiotics are given. The significance of mycoplasma in infertility must still be clarified but this remains a significant area of investigation.

Cigarette smoking is a far from benign habit. We are all acutely aware of the association of cigarette smoking with lung cancer, respiratory diseases, and cardiovascular diseases. Cigarette smoking can also affect ovarian function. A woman who smokes appears to develop several ovarian problems that may be associated with infertility. We also know that cigarette smoking is associated with earlier menopause. At a time when childbearing is being postponed to a later time in life, it becomes critical to take all the steps we can to ensure that the later years of reproduction are as free from compromise as possible. There is also evidence that cigarette smoking may produce serious damage to the developing embryo. Regular cigarette smoking may injure the fetus in several ways. Some are immediately apparent; others more subtle and insidious. Each puff of cigarette smoke introduces carbon monoxide and nicotine into the mother's circulation. This combination reduces blood flow to the fetus, which, on a repeated basis, may very well be damaging. Nicotine crosses the placenta to the developing fetus, affecting its cardiovascular and respiratory systems. A woman need not smoke directly to affect her fetus. She can inhale the cigarette smoke of others around her (so-called passive smoking) and be exposed to many of the same adverse substances that the smoker is exposed to.

A woman attempting pregnancy must consider herself possibly pregnant during every cycle. Quite often the pregnancy is a product of great effort and for that reason must be considered a premium pregnancy. But *every* pregnancy should be considered a premium pregnancy, and women should avoid the use of alcohol, drugs, caffeine, and exposure to radiation and cigarette smoke as well.

THE PSYCHOLOGICAL ELEMENT

The fourth main category of causes of infertility is that of psychological causes. Though this may not be a significant problem at the outset of the infertility workup and treatment, psychological problems may become significant later on. Once a doctor identifies the problems of a particular couple and begins treatment, an effort is made to determine as precisely as possible when ovulation occurs so the couple may have intercourse at that time and maximize the probability of achieving pregnancy. Often the result is that the couple is sent home with a schedule of recommended times for sexual activity. Asking a man and a woman to have sexual intercourse, month after month, at precise, predetermined times places a great deal of stress on both partners. An activity that should represent the ultimate in human pleasure may be reduced to a mechanical act or even drudgery. As a result the man may be unable to ejaculate on the days required, or there is so much tension on the woman's part that penile entrance into her vagina becomes impossible. Stress, whether the result of the outside world such as business pressures and the like, or a result of attempting pregnancy, may affect both partners. A man's sperm count and motility may be reduced through his hormonal system. Or the ability to perform sexually may be hampered.

Severe stress may turn off the ovulatory mechanism. In a school dormitory, at the time of midterm and final examinations, many girls who have had regular menses suddenly find that they have missed their periods. This is usually a result of the turning off of ovulation under stress. Exactly the same thing may happen to a couple attempting pregnancy. Though the woman may never have had an ovulatory problem before, after other problems are corrected and a pregnancy is attempted, she may cease ovulating, thus adding an additional problem. Fortunately, as we'll see in Chapter 6, this can be treated, as many other ovulatory problems can be.

Stress may also affect the coordinated movement of the Fallopian tubes. Though this is much more controversial, it appears that under certain *very limited* circumstances tension may cause a lack of coordination of the movement of the tubes that allow the egg to be transported in one direction and the sperm in another. Proper tubal movement, pickup of the egg, and its movement toward the uterus may be hampered thus leading to infertility. As our knowledge of other factors in infertility increases, the number of times we fall back on the psychological cause as an explanation diminishes.

Telling people that they are actively causing their own infertility by worrying about their lack of success creates a self-defeating situation. It creates guilt where little or none may have existed before. Warning someone that she must not worry or else she will not become pregnant is like saying "Do not think about your breathing." After you warn people not to think in a certain manner, they cannot help thinking in precisely that manner. Other than heightening anxiety and making sexual performance difficult, it is not even clear that the psychological factor is truly important in most infertile couples.

GENETIC FACTORS

It is possible for the genetic material produced in an egg or a sperm cell to be defective, and in that case fertilization usually does not take place. A defective sperm cell rarely works and a defective egg usually cannot be fertilized. If fertilization does occur and a defective structure is produced, there is frequently an early miscarriage.

Repeated miscarriage, unrelated to hormonal and structural

problems in the woman, requires a genetic evaluation of both partners. Blood is drawn from both the man and woman and genetic studies are done on the cells obtained from these samples. Several weeks are required for this study. Unfortunately, genetic problems are not treatable at this time. However, given the information that can be obtained from genetic studies, the couple can plan their future realistically, based on more complete information.

WHEN NO CAUSE IS FOUND

The last category is that of infertility of undetermined cause. Presently this represents one of the greatest challenges to the infertility specialist. This category is composed of a small number of couples for whom all adequate studies have been completed without finding a reason for infertility. Note that I have not said that these patients are normal. These couples are not told "There is nothing wrong with you," or "It is all in your head so go home and keep trying." As long as a man and a woman cannot accomplish what other couples can, they cannot be thought of as having nothing wrong with them. It is just that our tests may not be sensitive enough or sophisticated enough to find the problem. We, the specialists in reproductive medicine, are not yet smart enough to know all the possible causes and cures of infertility and, therefore, we do not know the answer for these couples. The one thing that is clear is that as the specialty of reproductive endocrinology and infertility advances, month by month, year by year, the percentage of couples with "infertility of undetermined cause" becomes smaller and smaller. Since we are not able to find the cause of this group's problems we are not able to treat them. Therefore, it is encouraging that as our knowledge expands, the number of people who fit into this category decreases and more and more couples are being helped.

Now that I have described the theoretical reasons for infertility, the next logical step is to determine which cause (or causes) applies to a particular couple. In the next chapter I discuss infertility testing.

CHAPTER 5
Infertility Tests

THE TESTS to determine the cause of childlessness at first seem like a meaningless obstacle course that a couple must endure before a physician can give them the reason for their problem and begin to help them. The procedures become even more difficult to endure because frequently, by necessity, they are distributed over several weeks or months. Some tests are rather uncomfortable, most are not. Understanding why each procedure must be done and why it must be done at a certain time makes it a bit easier to tolerate. In this chapter I will discuss the most commonly used tests in an infertility evaluation, tell you how they are done, why they are done, why they are done at specific times, and what kind of information you can expect from them.

GENERAL TESTS

One of the most helpful studies done during the course of an infertility evaluation is not a sophisticated biochemical test. It does not require the use of expensive equipment. It is simple, painless, and does not take weeks to provide information. It is accomplished simply by talking with your doctor and answering some detailed questions. The initial interview with your physician allows him or her to obtain an extensive history from both of you. This history will provide basic clues to the origin of the infertility.

An important first question is "How long have you been attempting pregnancy?" I ask this to establish whether or not you have had a sufficient opportunity to achieve pregnancy. Eighty percent of those couples who will establish a pregnancy do so in one year. Based on this, medical science has agreed that if a couple has had regular intercourse for one year without achieving pregnancy, the man and woman have an infertility problem. By regular intercourse, I mean sexual activity at least every other day at the time of ovulation, for twelve months.

The second general group of questions involves past reproductive history. Has the woman ever been pregnant before? If she has, how did the pregnancies end—with the birth of a live, healthy baby at term or with a miscarriage? Has the man ever fathered a pregnancy? Were these pregnancies with the same partner as now or with someone else?

Specific questions directed toward each of you will explore the possible reasons for infertility more completely. For the woman: Do you have regular periods with cramping? If you do, the chances that you are ovulating are very high. Irregular, painless menses that come as a complete surprise are usually not associated with ovulation. Though this is not an absolute rule, it does indicate some possibilities that require particular attention in the infertility studies. Do you feel one-sided, lower abdominal cramping or discomfort around midcycle? This is called *mittelschmertz* and refers to the cramping feeling associated with ovulation. The regular presence of mittelschmertz is further indication that ovulation is probably occurring. Many women who ovulate regularly never feel this discomfort. The presence of mittelschmertz makes the occurrence of ovulation likely, while its absence means nothing.

The history obtained by the physician can rule out major causes of Fallopian tube scarring. Have you ever had abdominal surgery of any kind? Have you ever had gonorrhea or any pelvic infections? Did you have an infection of your uterus after an abortion or the birth of your last child? Though you may have no reason for tubal adhesions based on past history, adhesions may still be present. The history obtained by your physician can only tell him that certain things are likely, not that they do not exist at all.

The male partner is questioned about previous surgery to his penis or testes. Did you ever have an infection of the testes? Did you have mumps as an adult? Have you ever had gonorrhea? Your doctor will ask about occupational or environmental factors. Is your job or life in general a stressful one? Are you exposed to pesticides, paints, solvents, cleaning fluids, high temperatures, or radiation? All of these factors may decrease sperm production and motility.

What kind of underwear do you wear? Anything that increases the temperature of the testes, such as briefs or tight tennis shorts, will provide an unfavorable environment for sperm production, resulting in a lowered sperm count and motility. Occasionally, changing underwear from briefs to boxer shorts can make a significant improvement in sperm quality—but it takes about ninety days for an improvement to be seen. Tight underwear is not the only way of elevating the temperature of the testes. Sitting for long periods of time as an office desk worker, cab driver, or truck driver will accomplish the same thing.

Do you use any medication? Tranquilizers and drugs used to treat high blood pressure are two examples of drugs that can decrease sperm production or make ejaculation (the release of sperm by the penis) difficult. Do you use lubricants, such as petroleum jelly, when having intercourse? Almost all lubricants decrease sperm movement and therefore make the sperm cells less effective.

Are you on any special diets? An unusually drastic reduction in calories can affect sperm quality. Other questions to investigate a history of diabetes, thyroid disease, and adrenal diseases in each member of the couple and their families are asked.

It would be impossible to review all that a complete infertility history covers. These examples are presented so that you can see what information can be obtained simply by talking with your doctor and answering questions.

The initial interview is more than an opportunity for the doctor to obtain information. It is also an excellent time for you to ask questions. This is important because only by doing this will you have an opportunity to satisfy your curiosity and expose your fears. It is very rare for the facts to be as frightening as the fears carried by most couples. The interview should not be a one-way interrogation, with the physician asking the questions and the couple answering them. Rather, this first meeting should be an easy interchange among all three people. Each member of the group asks and answers questions. In this way a rapport can be established and the basis for further and continuous communication and proper treatment is established.

Because nervousness in the physician's office—a common, normal reaction—can make it difficult to think of the questions that have been plaguing you for weeks and months, it is helpful to write down your questions and thoughts before coming for the initial interview. It may also be helpful to take notes in the doctor's office to help you remember instructions and responses to your key questions. Though some people feel self-conscious about doing this, there is no reason to feel that way. You are going to a physician for help and you should do everything possible to move toward success.

Following the interview the doctor conducts a complete physical examination. Routine screening blood tests are frequently obtained on the first visit. It is only during subsequent visits that specialized infertility studies are carried out.

SPECIALIZED TESTS

Specialized infertility tests can be divided into four general categories. The first is an evaluation of the male. The second is the determination of whether or not ovulation occurs in the female. The third is the determination of the architecture of the woman's reproductive system. And the fourth is an evaluation of the sperm within the female reproductive tract.

The entire workup should be completed, even if a reason for infertility is discovered in the process of evaluating the couple. In some cases there might be more than one reason for infertility. Because a woman is not ovulating, does not mean she could not also have an obstruction of one or both Fallopian tubes and/or her husband may have poor sperm. If a doctor stopped the evaluation at the point where it was discovered that the woman is not ovulating and treated her for that alone, the other problems would not be discovered and pregnancy still would not occur. Thus, barring some special circumstances, the entire infertility evaluation should be completed regardless of the findings during the progress of the workup. In medicine, as in many other things, no rules are absolute.

Evaluating the Man

Evaluation of the man is relatively simple. He is asked to produce a semen specimen by masturbation, deposit it into a clean glass jar, and deliver it to a laboratory for evaluation within two to three hours of producing the specimen. If he is unable to masturbate, the specimen may be collected by having sexual relations and withdrawing the penis from the vagina just prior to the release of sperm, and then releasing the sperm into a glass container. Where withdrawal of the penis cannot be accomplished in time, a special plastic condom may be used. The sperm collected this way may then be brought to the laboratory for analysis. Unfortunately, the materials out of which condoms are constructed and sometimes the chemicals used to line condoms may affect the sperm and can damage or kill some of the sperm cells, producing an artificially poor specimen. If the choice is between getting a specimen by this manner or no way at all then the use of a condom may be making the best of a poor situation.

In the laboratory the total volume of the fluid is measured. The number of sperm cells per unit volume is counted and reported to the doctor. The sperm cells themselves are then studied. Not all sperm produced are of normal shape nor are all the sperm cells moving. It is only the normal, moving sperm cells that are capable of producing pregnancy. The moving sperm cells are described as *motile* sperm cells. After the sperm are counted, a slide is made and both the percentage of all sperm cells that are moving and the percentage of all sperm cells of normal shape are recorded. The physician thus receives a report stating the volume of fluid, the number of sperm cells per unit volume of fluid, the percentage of normal forms seen, and the percentage of motile, or moving, forms seen. All these factors are important in determining the ability of the male partner to produce a pregnancy. Different laboratories have different "normal" values depending on their particular counting and dilution techniques. It is important when reading a given laboratory report to know what the normal values are for that particular laboratory.

An average for the general population is a count of more than 40 million cells per millimeter with a motility of greater than 50 percent, and 50 percent of those sperm cells will be of normal shape. We can also make certain of those sperm cells will be of normal shape. We can also make certain judgments about the probability of pregnancy associated with these various numbers.

Some men with semen analyses well within normal limits still fail to father a child even with several different partners of previously proven fertility. Semen analysis simply does not give us all the information that we would wish. There is something missing.

The best test would be to take the sperm cells and put them right next to a human egg and see whether or not the spermatozoa were capable of fertilizing eggs. However, creating new embryos simply for the purpose of testing sperm cells is neither ethically acceptable nor technically possible. And so some other means for the assessment of sperm cells was looked for. One suggestion was to take eggs from some other species and treat them in a way that they might be able to be fertilized by human sperm. Such fertilized eggs would not go on to form some strange new organism but would be a test of how well the human sperm cells could fertilize. This is exactly what has been done with hamster eggs. By collecting oocytes (eggs) from hamsters and pretreating them in a certain way, it is possible for human sperm cells to fertilize these eggs. This test is called a *hamster oocyte in vitro fertilization* study, sometimes simply referred to as a *hamster study*.

At first, there was reason to believe that this was the final assessment of the male in reproductive medicine. This was the test that was going to tell us if sperm cells of a specific individual were capable of fertilizing egg cells. Newer data derived from test-tube baby procedures using human eggs question the reliability of the hamster test. Investigators have found men whose sperm did not demonstrate the ability to fertilize on hamster study but fertilized their wives' eggs during *in vitro* fertilization. Doing a hamster study to evaluate how well human sperm cells can fertilize can be misleading. Further development of this study may make it more reliable in the future. At this time, a judgment that a male is unable to fertilize human eggs on the basis of a hamster study appears to be unreliable.

The semen sample should also be checked for fructose levels. Fructose is a sugar the epididymis adds to the seminal fluid. A semen analysis that shows no sperm does not indicate whether the testis has failed to produce sperm or if normal sperm has been produced but cannot reach the penis because of an obstruction in the path to the penis. Analysis of the sample for fructose levels can help in differentiating between these two conditions. If no sperm are present but fructose is found we know that the epididymis is present in that patient and that its secretions have found their way up through the vas deferens, out through the urethra and the opening of the penis. If, on the other hand, no fructose is found, then we must consider a possibility of a congenital absence of the epididymis or an obstruction of the vas deferens. In this case it is possible that the testis is making sperm but because of an obstruction in its pathway, it cannot reach the penis and the outer world.

To further evaluate the man who is *azospermic*, that is, produces no sperm, the physician will consider removing a small sliver of the testis and studying it under the microscope. This procedure, called a *testicular biopsy*, is done under anesthesia and is used to determine whether or not an azospermic man is indeed producing sperm within his testes. If the doctor sees sperm cells on biopsy then there is an obstruction somewhere in the system connecting the testes to the penis. If the doctor sees no sperm cells then he or she will pay particular attention to a microscopic examination of the structures involved. Frequently, this will give clues to appropriate drug treatment that may help to improve a man's fertility.

Another test sometimes used to evaluate an azospermic man is an X-ray procedure to examine the pathway from the testes to penis to assure that it is open and unobstructed. The procedure, called *vasography*, is done by putting a tube into the vas deferens and injecting dye. If X-rays are taken at this time, the path of the dye through this structure can be seen and a point of obstruction, if it exists, pinpointed. These studies are reserved for severely oligospermic or azospermic men—those who have very little or absolutely no sperm in their ejaculates.

If an endocrine problem is being considered, blood is drawn for FSH and LH levels and for thyroid studies, and a twenty-four–hour urine sample may be collected for 17-hydroxysteroid, 17-ketosteroid, and pregnantriol levels.

Evaluating the Woman

The second group of tests involve the woman. These include studies that determine whether or not ovulation occurs. If we were to sit down and attempt to devise a way of figuring out if a woman is making eggs it would be helpful to figure out something that happens after the production and the release of an egg that is not found under ordinary circumstances. When we think about it, it becomes apparent that the hormone progesterone is produced after ovulation and is not produced before or without ovulation. Progesterone has the ability to raise the temperature of a woman and to cause certain changes in the lining of the uterus.

The simplest test for ovulation is simply taking the temperature, orally or rectally, the first thing in the morning, before getting out of bed, before beginning any activity. This is important because any movement after arising requires the release of energy by the body and therefore elevates the resting temperature. The temperature recorded first thing in the morning, before any activity, is called the *basal body* temperature. It is more uniform and will reflect the presence or absence of progesterone more clearly.

Each morning, the first thing upon arising, the woman measures her temperature and records it on a temperature chart known as a Basal Body Temperature chart next to the particular day of her cycle, calling the first day of her menses cycle day one.

When all the dots on the temperature chart are connected, if ovulation has occurred, that part of the temperature chart following ovulation will show an elevation and a flat, straight line until just prior to menses. With the onset of menses or perhaps a day earlier, the woman's temperature will fall back to her preovulatory levels. It is important to realize that the level of the temperature does not reflect the amount of progesterone produced. Nor can anyone determine precisely when ovulation occurs from the temperature curve. One merely has the impression of a particular interval of several days during which time ovulation probably has occurred. (See Figure 5.1.)

Classically, the temperature curve around the time of ovulation shows a dip, then a gradual rise and a plateau lasting approximately fourteen days. Ovulation may occur anywhere from the dip to the rise, to the beginning of the plateau. It is impossible to determine while the curve is occurring, that is, during the menstrual cycle, exactly what day ovulation has occurred based on the shape of the curve.

The advantages of the basal body metabolism chart are that measuring temperature is an inexpensive and painless procedure. However, the test is basically a crude one and the information generated somewhat unreliable. There are women who have demonstrated that they ovulate by various tests but who do not produce a temperature curve consistent with ovulation. There are others for whom the rising part of the curve occurs over a several-day period. You need not get terribly disturbed if your own basal body temperature curve does not resemble the classic ones in the textbooks. The only information you should attempt to get from a temperature curve is preliminary information confirming that ovulation occurs and to determining the approximate time, within a several-day period, that it occurred in past cycles.

Progesterone causes certain changes in the structure of the tissue lining the uterus. The changes are so regular and predictable that it is possible to look at a piece of tissue taken from the lining of the uterus and by examining at its structure, determine how

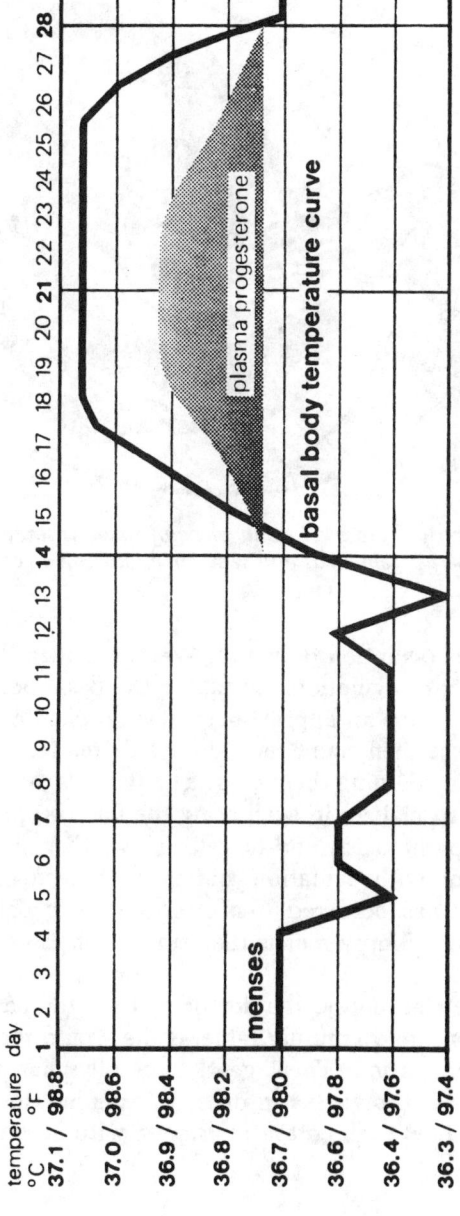

Figure 5.1 Basal body temperature. *When a woman's temperature is measured immediately upon awakening and is charted according to the day of the menstrual cycle, the result is a basal body temperature curve. The hormone progesterone, which is produced only after ovulation, makes a woman's basal temperature rise. Thus, if ovulation has occurred, the basal body temperature curve will show a rise and a plateau after ovulation. Note that the rise and fall in basal temperature somewhat parallels the rise and fall of progesterone levels.*

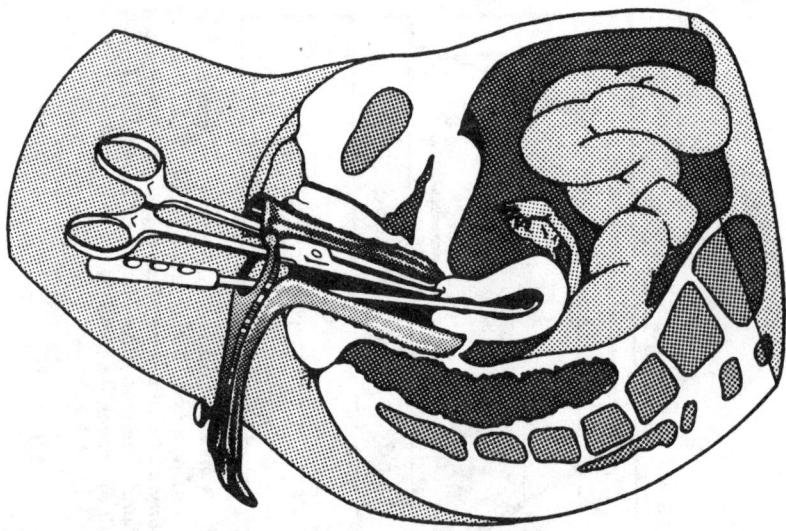

Figure 5.2 *Endometrial biopsy. A small piece of tissue is scraped from the lining of the uterus, removed, and sent for microscopic evaluation.*

many days earlier ovulation occurred. We can utilize this as a more accurate test of ovulation. By taking the basal body temperature curve we have an approximate idea of when a woman releases an egg. We then count several days thereafter and take a sample of the tissue lining the uterus. The tissue is then sent to a physician who specializes in evaluating the microscopic structure of tissue, a pathologist, and he tells us whether or not the tissue is consistent with ovulation and if so, how many days earlier ovulation has occurred. This procedure is called an *endometrial biopsy.* Biopsy means the removal of tissue for examination.

For an endometrial biopsy, the doctor will ask the patient to position herself on the examining table as she would for an ordinary pelvic examination. Then, gently, the physician will insert a speculum into the vagina in order to examine the cervix. The vagina is cleaned with cotton moistened with an antiseptic

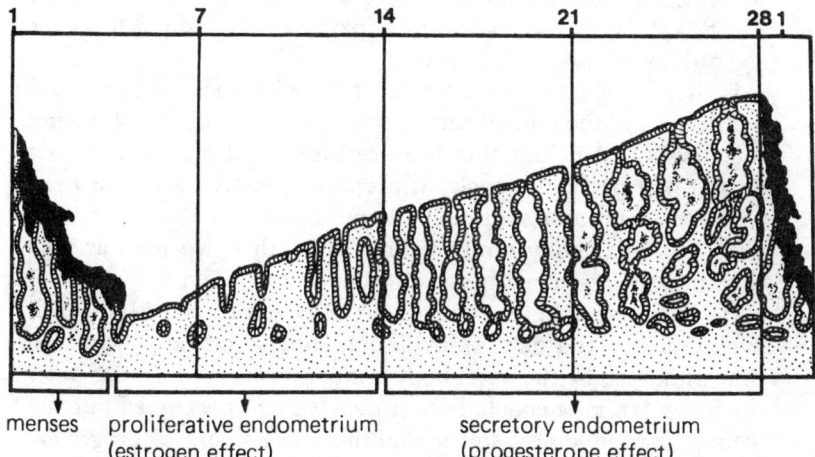

menses   proliferative endometrium   secretory endometrium
(estrogen effect)   (progesterone effect)

Figure 5.3 *The lining of the uterus. The endometrium, the tissue lining the uterus, has one structure before ovulation (proliferative endometrium) and a different structure after ovulation (secretory endometrium). The secretory endometrium is a result of progesterone action in the endometrium. Since progesterone is only produced after ovulation, the presence of secretory endometrium is presumptive evidence that ovulation has occurred.*

liquid. Up to this point the sensations felt by the woman are almost identical to those associated with a routine Pap smear examination. Next, the physician will grasp the cervix with a clamp to stabilize the uterus for the biopsy itself. The patient will feel a sudden, sharp pinching sensation lasting for several seconds; this is usually well tolerated because the discomfort is so brief. Next your doctor inserts a thin metal tube, called a *curette*, through the cervix into the uterine cavity. The doctor quickly withdraws the curette, scraping off a piece of the lining of the uterus. (See Figures 5.2 and 5.3) As the instrument is withdrawn the woman feels a cramp like a strong menstrual cramp. The discomfort lasts for about one minute and then dissipates over the next two to three minutes. The patient may experience some vaginal staining for up to several days following the biopsy. For this she may use a sanitary napkin or a tampon, whichever she ordinarily use for her menses.

If the pathologist's report returns showing that ovulation did not occur and the temperature curve confirms this, the physician may begin to conclude that the woman has not ovulated at least during that particular cycle. If the report comes back consistent with ovulation and ovulation has occurred at a time consistent with the basal body temperature curve, then we may assume that an egg has indeed been released.

It is also possible that the report may return consistent with ovulation but the date of ovulation differs radically from the time estimated by the basal body temperature curve. In this case, the physician may conclude that ovulation has occurred but the woman is producing a lower than normal amount of progesterone. The biopsy can also tell the physician whether or not a chronic infection of the uterine cavity, such as tuberculosis, might exist.

The advantage of the endometrial biopsy is that it provides data that is much more reliable than the basal body temperature in terms of confirming or denying that ovulation occurs. Its disadvantage is that it is somewhat uncomfortable, although it should be easily tolerated in most cases. And if the patient has become pregnant during that particular cycle, there is a small chance in taking the endometrial biopsy that pregnancy may be interrupted, causing a miscarriage.

Another test for ovulation is to measure progesterone levels directly. This can be done simply by drawing blood from the woman's arm at a time of her cycle when the progesterone levels should be highest. The advantages of this test are that it is less uncomfortable than an endometrial biopsy and still gives excellent information about whether or not ovulation has occurred. The test also provides direct and accurate information about progesterone levels following ovulation. It appears to be the best way to diagnose a luteal phase deficiency. The disadvantage is that the test provides no information about the normality or abnormality of the tissue lining the uterine cavity. Only an endometrial biopsy can provide this information. Many infertility specialists use both the endometrial biopsy and a plasma progesterone level done at the midluteal phase (about one week after the expected ovulation) to investigate ovulation. (See Figure 5.4.)

Testing for Structural Problems in Women

The third group of infertility tests are those that study the structure of the uterus and Fallopian tubes. It is impossible for a woman to achieve pregnancy by ordinary means without having at least one open tube through which an egg might be picked up and in which fertilization of that egg can take place. Repeated loss of pregnancy may occur if the uterine cavity is distorted or abnormal in shape. If the uterine cavity is so distorted that most of the cavity is absent, pregnancy may never occur at all. Thus, evaluation of the uterine cavity and both Fallopian tubes is very important.

This aspect of fertility may be evaluated indirectly through the *Rubin's insufflation test*, more directly by a specialized X-ray procedure called a hysterosalpingogram, or most directly and accurately by *endoscopy*. Endoscopy is a technique of directly examining the structure and working of the human body by inserting a small telescope into different parts of the body. The three types of endoscropy—hysteroscopy, culdoscopy, and laparoscopy—will be discussed later in this chapter.

The principle behind the Rubin's insufflation test is simple. If you take a certain amount of gas and use it to inflate a balloon, as the balloon expands the pressure inside will build up. If a machine that draws a graph of the increasing pressure is attached to the balloon, you would get a curve of a certain shape. If the same balloon had two holes in it and the same amount of gas were pumped into it, the pressure produced in the balloon would be less. As the gas is pumped in at one end some of it would leak out of the balloon through the two holes. The curve made by the machine would be of different shape than when the balloon had no holes. This is precisely the principle of the Rubin's test. A pressure tube, connected to a machine which records pressure, is connected to the cervix and carbon dioxide gas is allowed to slowly enter the uterine cavity. If the woman has two

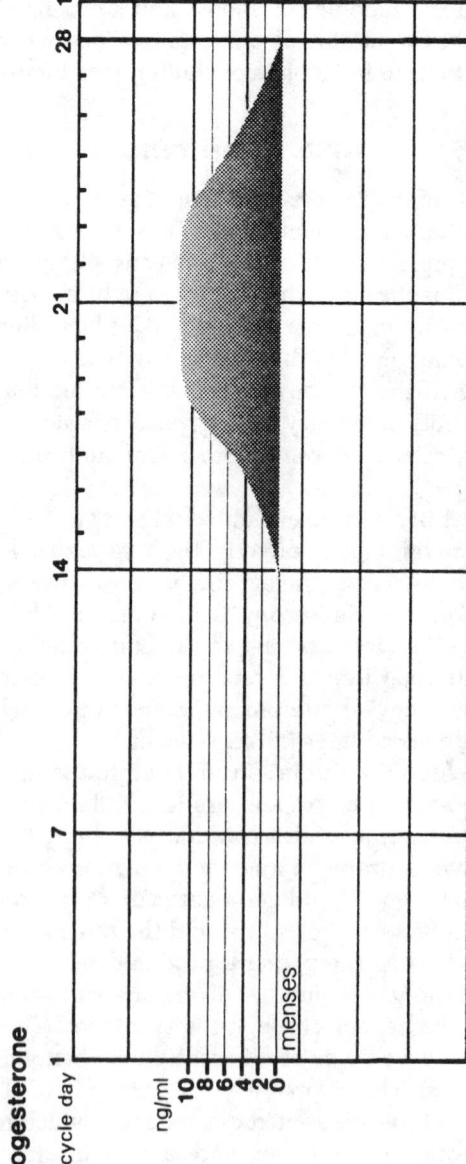

Figure 5.4 *Changes in plasma progesterone during the cycle. After ovulation the blood level of progesterone gradually increases, reaches its maximum between cycle days 20 and 23, and then gradually diminishes. Progesterone is produced only after ovulation. Thus, finding a significant blood level of this hormone is presumptive evidence of ovulation. This is best done between cycle days 19 and 24.*

open Fallopian tubes (that is, the channel within the tube is not blocked), as the gas flows into the uterine cavity some of it will leak out through the tubes. The gas will flow out into the abdominal cavity and irritate her diaphragm. Strangely enough, when the diaphragm is irritated the patient does not feel abdominal pain but shoulder pain. So if carbon dioxide gas leaks out of the uterine cavity through open Fallopian tubes, the patient will feel shoulder pain. As the machine records the pressure in the uterine cavity a curve is drawn; the pressure within the uterine cavity does not rise as rapidly as it would if none of the gas had leaked out. If, on the other hand, both tubes have been closed because of surgery or inflammation, then the carbon dioxide placed within the uterine cavity would not leak out. The patient would feel no shoulder pain and the pressure within the uterine cavity would build up very, very rapidly. The result would be a graph with a characteristic shape.

The advantage of the Rubin's test is that it can be done in the physician's office with no exposure to X-rays. The disadvantage is that the information is not terribly accurate. The Rubin's test offers general information as to whether there is at least one Fallopian tube open or closed. The doctor cannot determine anything about the shape of the uterine cavity, whether one tube is open and the other closed or both tubes are partially open. If both tubes are closed, the test offers no information as to where in the Fallopian tube the obstruction is.

If the test is normal, a hysterosalpingogram is still done to investigate the contour of the uterine cavity and to rule out the possibility of adhesions to the Fallopian tube. If the test is abnormal, indicating a possible obstruction of the Fallopian tube, an X-ray is still done to confirm the findings of the Rubin's test and to help locate the obstruction. Because any finding of the Rubin's test still requires hysterosalpingogram for further information, many physicians have stopped using the Rubin's test.

The word "hysterosalpingogram" is so long and complicated that it frequently makes people run and hide. The very sound of the word conjures up visions of a grotesque procedure designed to test the limits of human endurance. But, like so many words in medicine, it is composed of smaller words that describe exactly

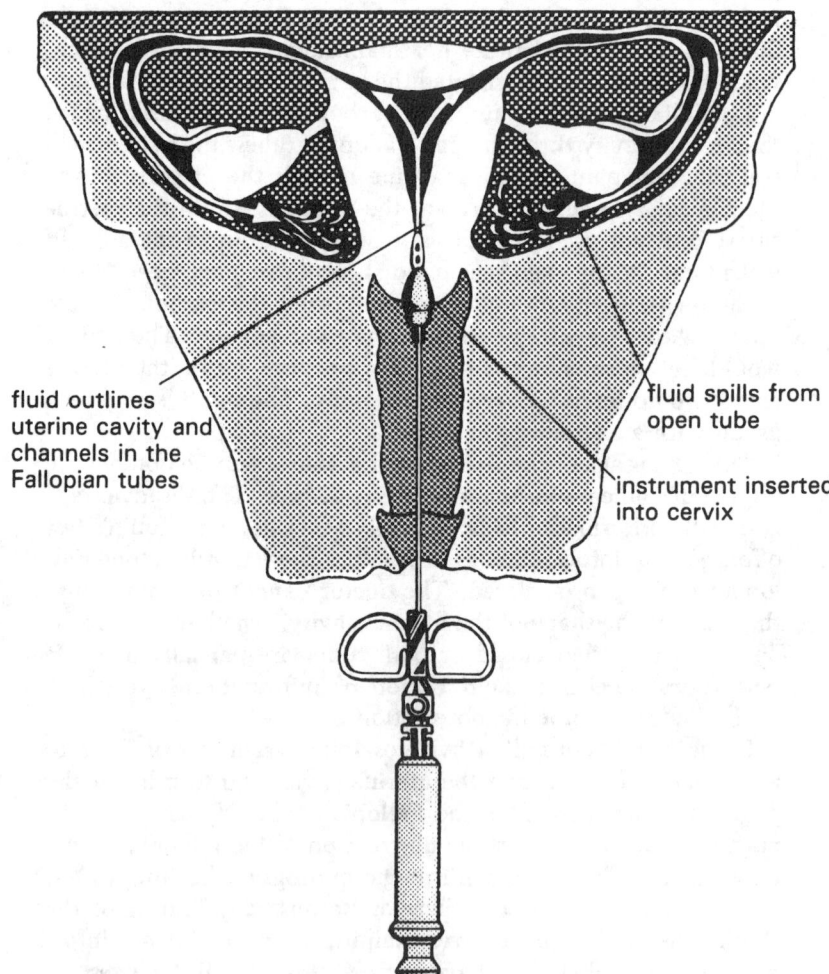

fluid outlines
uterine cavity and
channels in the
Fallopian tubes

fluid spills from
open tube

instrument inserted
into cervix

Figure 5.5 *Hysterosalpingogram. By injecting a fluid which can be seen on X-ray, one is able to take pictures of the cavity of the uterus and the tubes.*

what the procedure is designed to do. *Hystero* refers to the uterus. *Salpingo* refers to the Fallopian tubes. The *gram* part of it describes a picture. The result is a word meaning a "picture of the uterus and tubes," which is exactly what you want to have to evaluate a woman for infertility.

A woman goes to a radiologist's suite and lies on an X-ray table. A doctor inserts a tube with a rubber gasket into the cervix and into the uterine cavity. The tube is connected to a syringe containing a liquid dye that can be seen on X-ray.

An X-ray can show bony structures but soft, muscular structures such as the uterus and tubes will not show up. Gently pushing the plunger down on the syringe forces the dye to go through the metal tube into the uterine cavity. By taking X-rays at this time the physician can see the outline of the dye which has filled the cavity. The result is a silhouette of the uterine cavity. As the dye completely fills the uterine cavity, it begins to pour out through the Fallopian tubes, filling the channels in the tubes and eventually pouring out the ends of the tubes. If there is an obstruction in the tube, the dye will stop at that point, and the doctor can locate the point of obstruction. Something projecting into the uterine cavity, such as a fibroid (a benign tumor), or extending into the uterine cavity, such as a septum, a fibroid on a stalk, or a polyp, will be seen on the X-ray. As you can see, the hysterosalpingogram is a very helpful procedure and, short of endoscopy, which I discuss below, provides the greatest amount of information about the internal structure of a woman's reproductive system. (See Figures 5.5, 5.6, 5.7, 5.8, and 5.9.)

As the fluid fills the uterine cavity during a hysterosalpingogram, the uterus becomes slightly stretched and the patient may feel some discomfort. The sensation is usually described as feeling like a moderate menstrual cramp and it lasts for about two to three minutes longer than the injecting of fluid. The whole period of discomfort lasts for about ten minutes and most women easily tolerate it.

The advantages of the hysterosalpingogram are that it provides the maximum amount of information about a woman's reproductive system short of endoscopy. Like all things, the hysterosalpingogram has its disadvantages. First, it is an X-ray procedure,

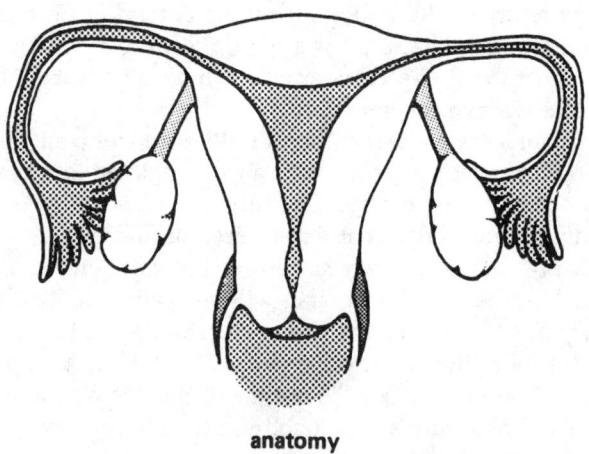

anatomy

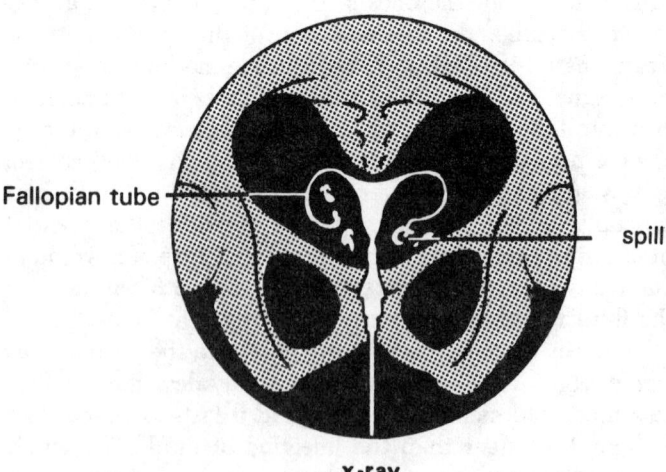

x-ray

Figure 5.6 *Normal hysterosalpingogram.*

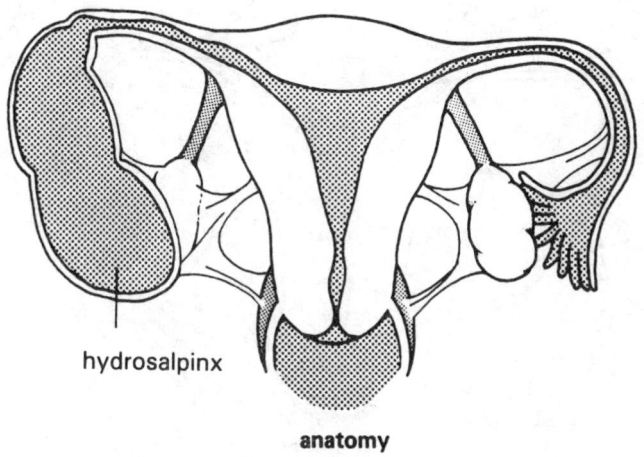

anatomy

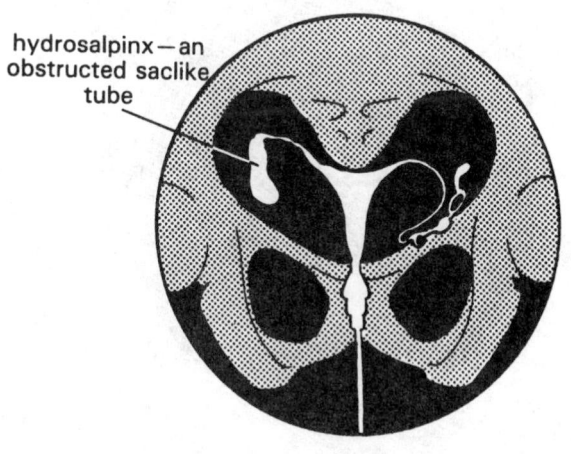

x-ray

Figure 5.7 *Hysterosalpingogram showing closure of one tube.*

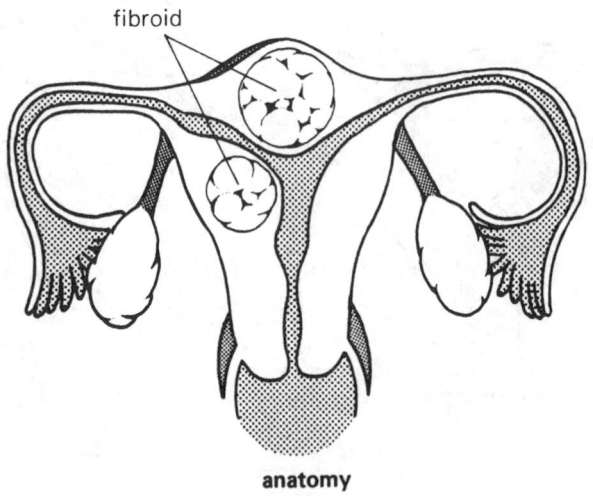

anatomy

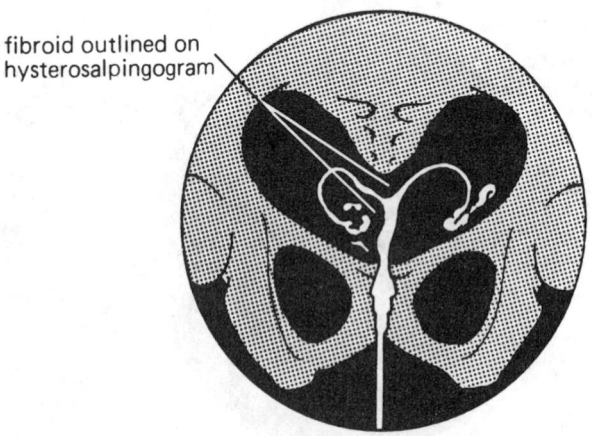

Figure 5.8 *Hysterosalpingogram showing distortion of the cavity of the uterus by fibroids.*

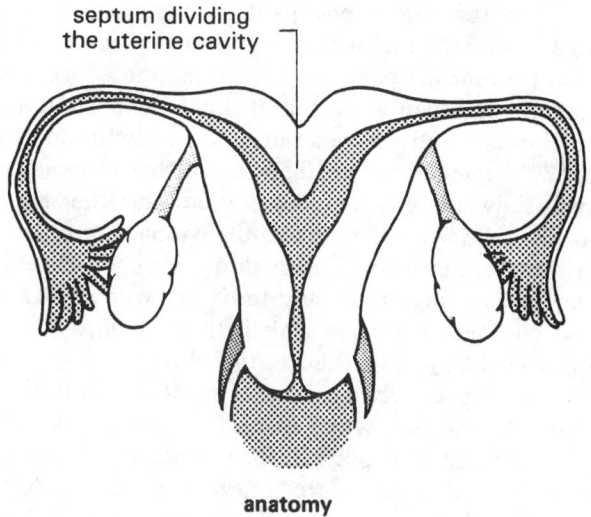

septum dividing
the uterine cavity

anatomy

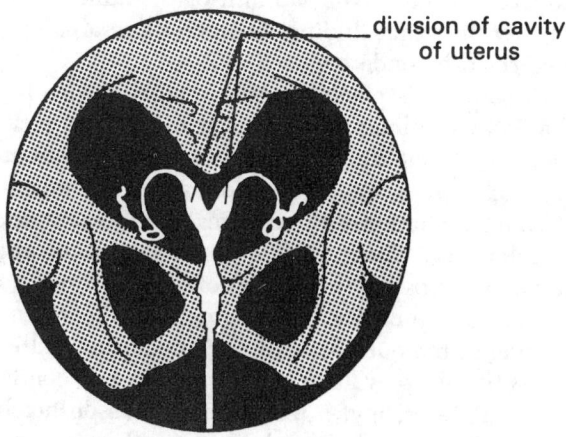

division of cavity
of uterus

Figure 5.9 *Hysterosalpingogram showing the upper portion of the cavity of the uterus divided by a septum (wall).*

subjecting the woman to radiation, although the dose is small and therefore the risk is not great. A hysterosalpingogram is scheduled during the first half of a woman's cycle—prior to ovulation—to prevent the possibility of irradiating a fertilized egg.

The second disadvantage is that it is not 100 percent accurate. While it is significantly more accurate than the Rubin's test, it is still only 70 percent accurate. This means that in some cases the X-ray will show there is something wrong in either the uterine cavity or the tube when there is nothing wrong. Conversely, there will be times when there is something wrong with either the uterus or the Fallopian tubes and the X-ray will appear normal. The most common reason for this is that the X-ray, by photographing the dye within the uterine cavity and the channels within the Fallopian tubes, shows the cavities within the organs rather than the tissues of which an organ is made. It fails to show its outside surfaces. It is possible for adhesions to be on the outside of the Fallopian tube distorting the tube and holding it in such a position that pickup of a released egg is impossible. Since the channel of the tube may be open and normal, the X-ray will appear normal, giving no hint of the adhesions on the outside. The result is that findings of the hysterosalpingogram should be confirmed by endoscopy.

Endoscopy is placing a telescopelike device into a portion of the body and looking through it to view a particular organ directly, without the aid of X-ray or any other indirect means. Generally, it is one of the most accurate diagnostic procedures available. There are three forms of endoscopy that are relevant to infertility. These are *hysteroscopy, culdoscopy* and *laparoscopy*. Hysteroscopy is a means of looking directly at the contents of the uterine cavity. Culdoscopy and laparoscopy are ways of looking at the outside surface of the uterus and Fallopian tubes, respectively, to evaluate their function and condition.

For hysteroscopy, a patient lies down on her back on an operating table under local or general anesthesia. The doctor slightly stretches the opening of the uterus, the cervix. Then the doctor inserts an instrument through the opening of the cervical canal and inflates the cavity of the uterus with either carbon dioxide gas or a clear fluid. When the uterus is distended so that the front and back walls are no longer touching, the doctor inserts a telescopelike device through the cervix into the uterine cavity. The physician then can look around and study the surfaces of the uterine cavity. The doctor can see the area where the Fallopian tubes join the uterus from the inside and study the actual opening of the tube on the inside of the uterus, and with special instruments and the hysteroscope, remove polyps, fibroids on stalks, and various other structures projecting into the uterine cavity that should not normally be there. The doctor can confirm the presence of a septum (wall) projecting into the uterine cavity and, under certain circumstances, can actually cut away the septum under hysteroscopic control. Using the hysteroscope, a doctor can locate and cut adhesions within the uterine cavity that may abnormally hold the front and back walls of the cavity together, thereby partially obliterating the cavity. (See Figure 5.10.)

The advantage of hysteroscopy is that it allows direct viewing of the contents of the uterine cavity. Under certain circumstances, a diagnosis made by a hysterosalpingogram can be confirmed by hysteroscopy and treatment accomplished using the hysteroscope. Removing an intrauterine polyp or a lost IUD are its most common uses. The doctor can treat the problem while looking directly at the problem area rather than using a blind procedure such as a dilatation and curettage (D and C). Most other endoscopic procedures associated with infertility are done under general anesthesia or very deep sedation. Hysteroscopy is most frequently done under general anesthesia but, under appropriate circumstances, may be done under only local anesthesia, thereby minimizing the risk to the patient. There are really very few risks with hysteroscopy.

There are times when it is very helpful to look at the Fallopian tubes directly. The methods I have described thus far of determining whether or not the tubes are open do not provide any detailed information about the outside of the Fallopian tubes and may not be very accurate. In an attempt to seek more precise information, the doctor may actually look at the Fallopian tube. To do this, anesthesia is administered and the doctor inserts a telescope into the abdomen and aims it toward the uterus, Fal-

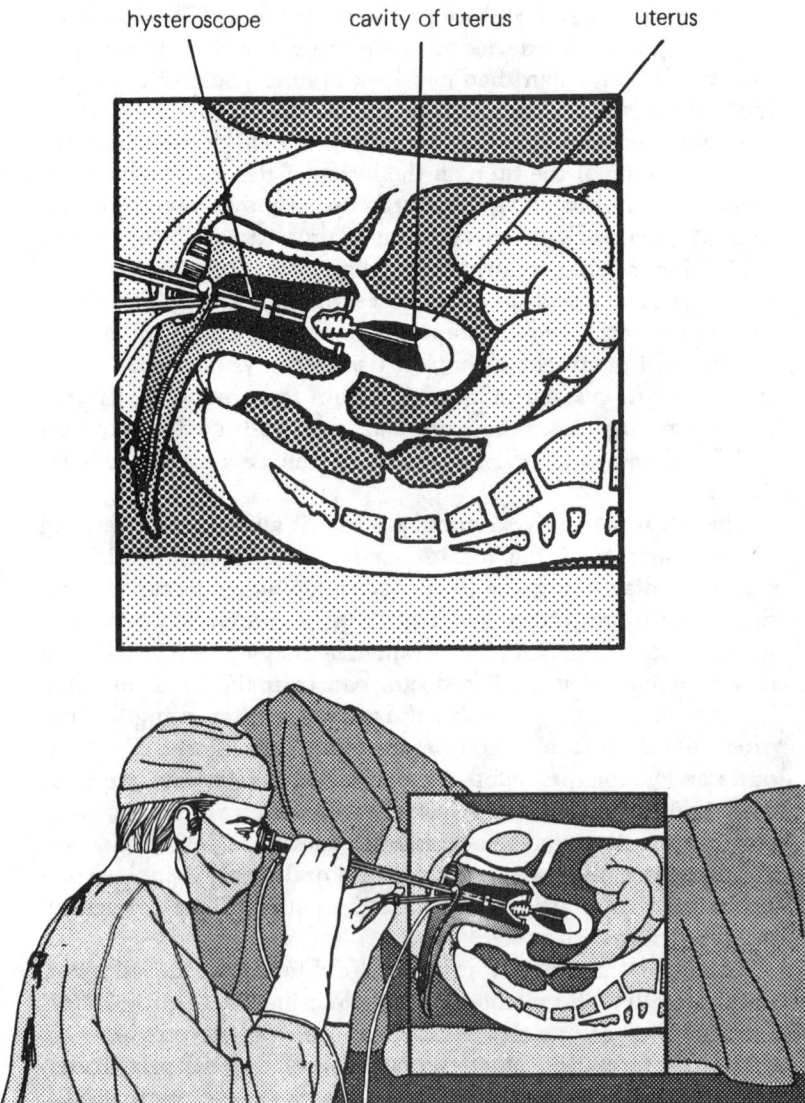

Figure 5.10 *Hysteroscopy. By inserting the hysteroscope into the vagina and through the cervix, the cavity of the uterus can be seen and evaluated.*

lopian tubes, and ovaries. Then the doctor fills the uterus with a dye solution in much the same way as for a hysterosalpingogram. Using the endoscope, the doctor can observe the dye solution filling and spilling out of the Fallopian tubes. This will confirm the degree to which the tubes are open or closed. Since the outside surface of the tubes may be seen, any adhesions that are present may be found. Under certain circumstances, the doctor may insert additional instruments and, if possible, cut adhesions. There may also be abnormalities of the ovaries or of the tubes. These may not be correctable using endoscopic instruments and regular abdominal surgery may be called for.

One of two routes may be selected for the insertion of the endoscope. The route chosen determines the kind of instrument used. Today, the most common route is through the umbilicus or belly button, hence the everyday term "belly-button surgery." The patient lies on an operating table on her back and is usually given general anesthesia. Under certain circumstances, local anesthesia will be used. The doctor makes a small incision in the lower edge of the umbilicus and then inflates the abdomen with carbon dioxide gas. The doctor inserts a telescopelike device called a *laparoscope* through the same incision in the umbilicus and studies the abdominal and pelvic contents. (See Figure 5.11.)

Another route involves the back wall of the vagina. As the illustration shows, by making a hole in the back wall of the vagina, just below the cervix, the doctor can easily enter the abdominal cavity (see Figure 5.12). This is called a culdoscopy. For this the patient will be deeply sedated and placed facedown on an operating table. Then her knees are brought toward her chest, so her vagina is directed back toward the surgeon. The doctor inserts instruments into the vagina to expose its back wall and makes a small incision just above the cervix. Through this incision the physician inserts a telescopelike device called a *culdoscope*. The doctor uses the culdoscope to study the back surface of the uterus, the Fallopian tubes, and ovaries as in laparoscopy. The doctor can see dye filling and spilling out of both tubes and can locate adhesions. By inserting instruments next to the culdoscope, the doctor can cut the adhesions and perform other

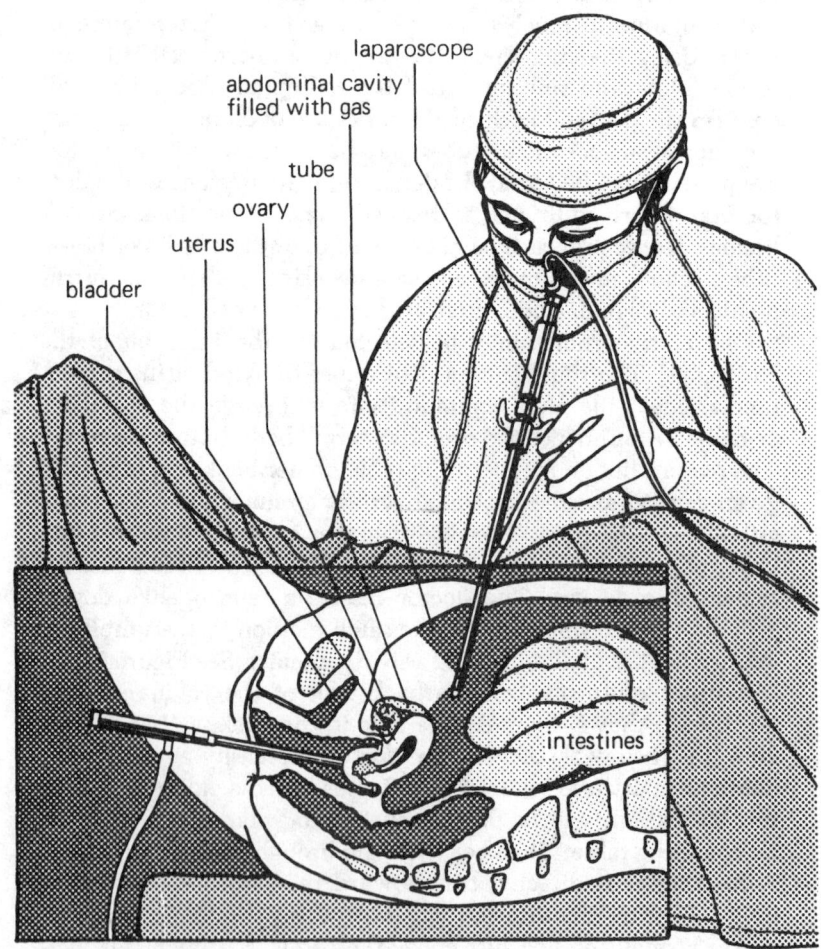

Figure 5.11 *Laparoscopy. By inserting the laparoscope through the navel of a woman, the physician can see and evaluate much of the contents of the abdomen, including the uterus, Fallopian tubes, and ovaries.*

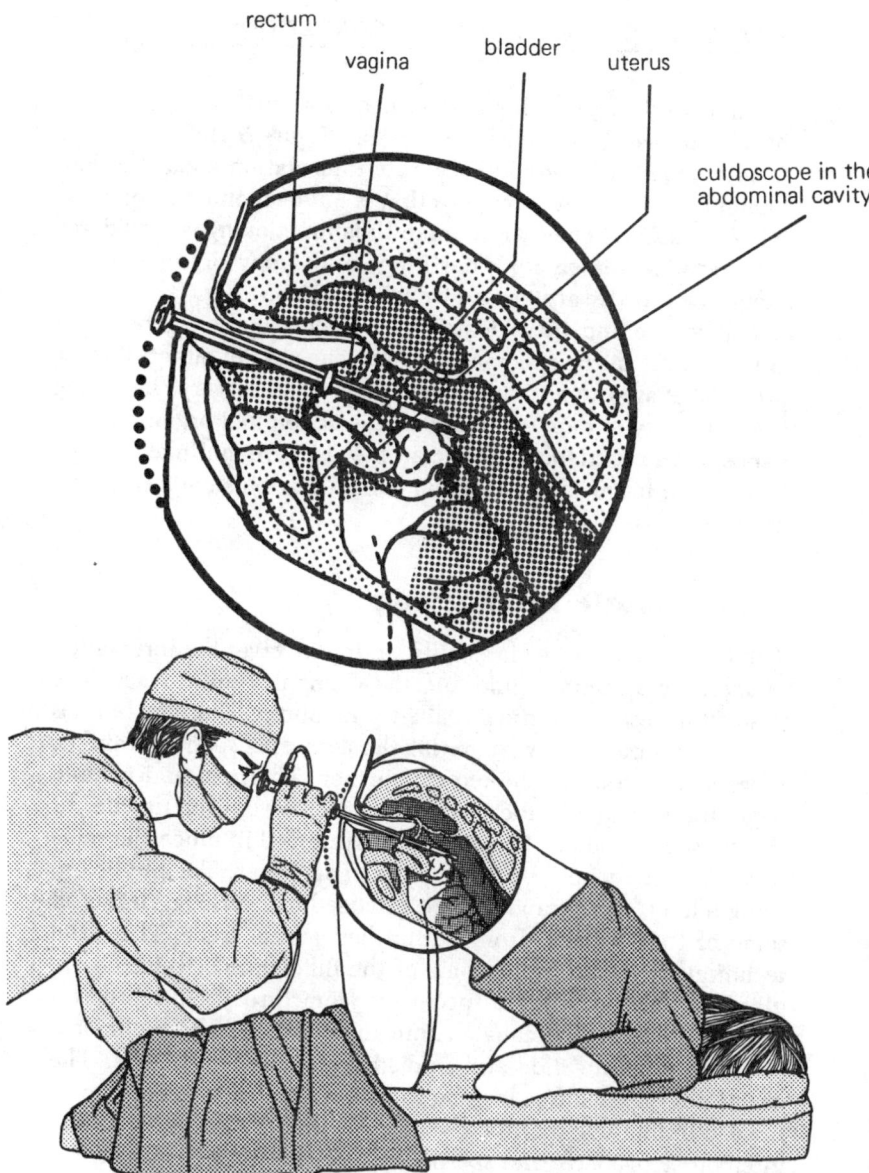

rectum

vagina

bladder

uterus

culdoscope in the abdominal cavity

Figure 5.12 *Culdoscopy. By inserting the culdoscope through the back of the vagina, the physician can see and evaluate the ovaries, Fallopian tubes, and the back of the uterus.*

limited surgical procedures. The need for further surgery may be ascertained during culdoscopy. (See Figure 5.12.)

Both procedures provide accurate information about the Fallopian tubes and any adhesions that is not available through any other means. Whenever Fallopian tube functioning is considered as a possible reason for infertility, culdoscopy or laparoscopy should be a necessary procedure in evaluation.

The couple and their doctor must decide if these procedures are advisable in their particular case. The risks of either of these procedures are the normal risks of abdominal surgery, including the possibility of damage to any of the abdominal organs. In the hands of an experienced physician the risks are minimal and the benefits, in terms of information gained and possible treatment, are enormous.

Male-Female Interaction

The fourth category of infertility testing involves the interaction of sperm and seminal fluid and the woman's genital tract. The postcoital test, sometimes called the Simms-Huhner test, is the most common means of testing the survival of sperm within the reproductive tract of the female partner. The man and woman have intercourse at midcycle and are seen several hours later at the physician's office. The woman is examined in much the same position as she would be for a routine Pap smear. The physician, using a long, thin strawlike tube attached to a syringe, draws off some of the secretion from within her genital tract. The usual technique involves taking some of the fluid from within the vagina and taking separate specimens from three points progressively further up the canal within the cervix. Each specimen is put on a separate slide and studied under the microscope. The examining physician is looking for live sperm cells in each specimen. Finding live sperm cells indicates that the couple is having intercourse properly and sperm are surviving in the woman.

In looking for a reason for infertility, nothing must be taken for granted. If the semen analysis demonstrates the presence of live sperm and the postcoital examination fails to show any sperm within the vagina, then—regardless of what the couple has told the doctor—the evidence indicates that the man is not delivering sperm into the woman's vagina, and there is a strong possibility of a problem with sexual technique.

If the postcoital test indicates live sperm within the vagina and cervix, the couple has been using a technique good enough to allow the delivery of live sperm into the vagina. If there are live sperm in the vaginal specimen and nonmoving sperm in the specimen taken from the cervix, there is something within the woman's reproductive tract that is killing off the sperm. There are several possible explanations.

There may be an allergic reaction where the woman's bodily defenses—which would ordinarily kill off foreign microorganisms—may falsely identify the sperm cells as a foreign organism and kill them. Another possibility is an infection in the woman's reproductive tract with a microorganism that provides a hostile environment for the sperm and causes the death of the sperm.

In the above descriptions it is assumed that there is a large quantity of watery, clear mucus in the cervix to support the life of the sperm cells for the test. Since this test is being done at midcycle, at the time that ovulation should occur, there should be cervical mucus present to act as a medium through which the sperm cells can swim on their way up through the cervix to the uterus, the Fallopian tube, and the egg.

It is possible for a woman to make a very small amount of cervical mucus or to make a cervical mucus so thick that instead of acting as a pathway for the sperm on its way up to the egg it acts as a barrier. If the latter is the case, in a postcoital examination the physician will find some live sperm in the vagina and a small or moderate amount of cervical mucus so thick that it is very difficult to withdraw it for microscopic study. When the specimen is put on the slide and studied under the microscope, few if any sperm cells are seen. If any are seen they are trapped in the mucus, unable to move. (See Figure 5.13.)

The postcoital test is relatively simple to do and can give a great deal of information. It can tell the physician about cervical mucus production and the survival of sperm within the woman's reproductive tract. It can also give your doctor a general idea of

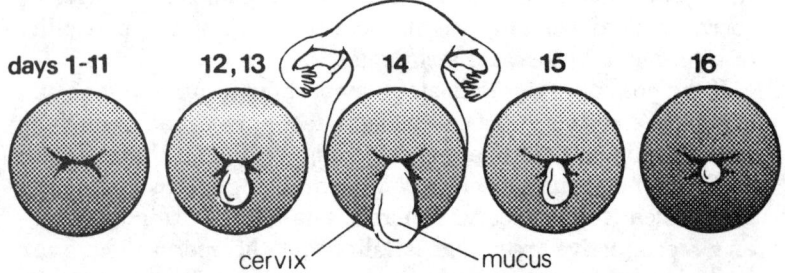

days 1-11   12, 13   14   15   16

cervix   mucus

Figure 5.13 *Cervical mucus. At the time of ovulation, the mucus produced by the cervix changes in volume and quantity. Before and after ovulation, there is a small amount of very thick, viscous mucus present. At ovulation and a day or so before and after, the volume of mucus increases and the quality changes to a clear watery liquid. Finding a large volume of clear watery cervical mucus is presumptive evidence of ovulation on or around the day of examination. Since such mucus allows sperm to enter the uterus and survive for a longer period, ovulation time is the best time to perform a postcoital test.*

the quality of sperm production. It involves no risk to either member of the couple.

Good cervical mucus production but poor survival of sperm cells within the cervical mucus indicates further testing is necessary. In most cases, the doctor should consider the possibility of an immunological problem. Both partners should be studied for antisperm antibodies.

Another possible explanation for poor sperm survival with adequate cervical mucus could be a microorganism infecting the reproductive tract. The doctor should also consider cultures of both the man's and the woman's reproductive tracts for T-strain mycoplasma, although this remains a controversial area of study.

If all of the basic studies outlined thus far have failed to demonstrate any reason for the couple's inability to have achieved a pregnancy, immunological studies of both members of the couple should still be performed. There is some incidence of antisperm antibodies in either partner even in the face of a normal postcoital test. Though this is a fairly uncommon situation, it must be considered when no other reason for infertility can be found.

Determining Time of Ovulation

For various reasons it would be helpful to know when an egg was actually released from a woman's ovary. It would make timing of intercourse simpler and would allow artificial insemination with greater precision. This is particularly important when artificial insemination is used with samples from a man with a very low sperm count. Such a man may be able to produce only one specimen of good quality throughout the time of ovulation. Therefore, it would be of great value to pick the best time to use this sample to allow the greatest probability of pregnancy. Basal body temperature charts are inexpensive but highly unreliable. At best, they can only bracket a time within four to five days that might include the time of ovulation. Other studies of ovulation, including ultrasound, are only slightly more reliable. Blood progesterone studies and endometrial biopsies determine that ovulation has probably occurred but do not precisely define when the egg was released.

In order to determine ovulation time, it would be helpful to find an event that always occurred on a regular basis just prior to the release of an egg. Such an event does occur and has been used recently in a new test to document the time of ovulation. Just prior to ovulation, the pituitary releases a massive amount of FSH and LH. This event is called the LH surge. Ovulation appears to occur within thirty-six hours of the LH surge. If there were a simple way to test for the LH surge, you could predict the exact time of ovulation.

After the pituitary produces the massive amount of hormone in the LH surge, the hormone spills out from the bloodstream into the urine. If you were to test the urine day after day, and if you could easily determine the amount of LH in the urine, then you should see that just prior to ovulation there is a sudden increase in the amount of LH in the urine. Using this test a woman could tell within twelve to twenty-four hours of the finding of a large amount of LH in the urine that ovulation should occur. A number of companies have released just such a test.

Urine samples are either tested with plastic paddles or test tubes impregnated with chemicals that will change color in the presence of LH. The color intensity is related to the amount of hormone present: the greater the amount of hormone, the darker the color change. Using such a test, one can determine the time of ovulation with great regularity. No test is foolproof, and sometimes ovulation will occur when the urine tests do not pick up any LH. The significance of the studies should be discussed with a physician but as a general guide these tests can be enormously helpful in determining a woman's most fertile time.

We perform tests, presumably, to find answers to questions. We hope to find out why a man and woman have been unable to produce a child. It is surprising that sometimes tests end up asking more questions rather than providing a definite answer. When basal body temperature, endometrial biopsy, and/or plasma progesterone levels show that ovulation is not occurring, we must then ask why. When sperm do not survive in the woman's reproductive tract, we must then ask why, because the answer to this question determines how easily the problem can be treated. If the woman has an obstruction of a Fallopian tube, we must ask where that obstruction is and how extensive it is because the probability of surgical success hinges on the answers.

Though a physician may lay out a plan of several tests at the initial consultation, other tests may prove necessary during the course of the workup. The trip from beginning to end may be long and at times seem complicated, but if you know why and how each test is done, the trip seems less involved and is easier to make. Make your physician your partner on this trip. Share your feelings and your fears with him or her. Try to understand your doctor's reasoning and conclusions at each point in the investigation. These tests are to be done *for* you and not *to* you. All three people—the man and the woman of the couple and the physician consulted—must have equal involvement.

Now that we have discussed the tests to be performed, let us progress to the treatment available.

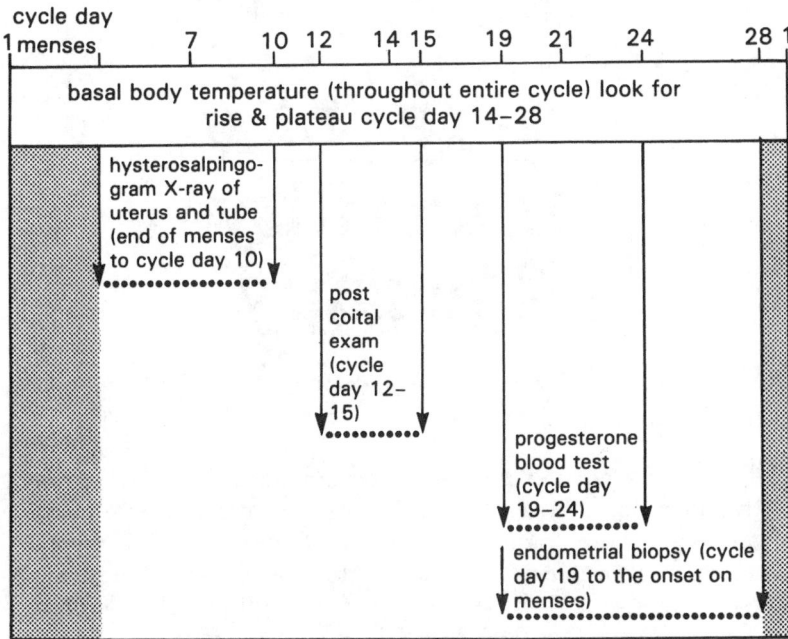

Figure 5.14 *Timing of infertility tests. A. Basal body temperature. This should be taken throughout the cycle. A sustained elevation in the curve in the second half of the cycle is consistent with ovulation.*
B. Hysterosalpingogram. This X-ray of the uterus and tubes should be taken after the end of menses and before the time of ovulation. To be sure to avoid ovulation, one frequently selects cycle day 10 or 11 as the last day for taking the X-ray.
C. Postcoital examination. This test is to evaluate how well sperm live in the cervical mucus of the woman being evaluated. Cervical mucus produced at the time of ovulation is best able to support the life of sperm. For this reason this test is usually scheduled between cycle days 12 and 15 of a 28-day cycle.
D. Progesterone blood test. Plasma progesterone is measured in a sample of blood drawn around the time of greatest progesterone production. This test is done between cycle days 19 and 24.
E. Endometrial biopsy. A sample of the tissue lining the uterus is removed and studied microscopically. If the sample was removed after ovulation, the tissue should have the structure of secretory endometrium. This tissue is best developed after cycle day 18. Thus, the biopsy or sampling of the endometrium is usually done between cycle day 19 and the onset of menses.

CHAPTER 6

Infertility Therapy

THIS ENTIRE chapter may easily be summarized by saying that treatment in each case must be applied to correct whatever abnormalities were found in the infertility investigation. If there is a structural problem, then the structure of the reproductive system must somehow be returned to normal. If a hormonal problem exists then that must be corrected.

A complete infertility evaluation must be finished before any treatment can begin. This evaluation cannot stop when one specific reason for infertility is found. It is possible that more than one cause for infertility may exist. It would be unfortunate if treatment were started after finding a single problem and, after six months or a year of unsuccessful treatment, the infertility evaluation were completed only to find that there was a second problem that was never even suspected. Infertility is a problem of couples, not of individuals, and the probability of success in the treatment of infertility is the total success possible after evaluation and treatment of both members of the couple.

FOR THE MAN

The first step in the man's evaluation is a semen analysis. If it is not normal, even after a second analysis for confirmation, your doctor will order a physical examination and laboratory studies.

X-ray studies and a testicular biopsy may be considered in some cases, as discussed in Chapter 5.

Drug Therapy

If the studies reveal that the man has a hormonal problem, treatment must be directed toward replacing or correcting what is missing. If the man has a pituitary malfunction resulting in low levels of the pituitary hormones FSH and LH, then he should be given FSH and LH. FSH is usually given in the form of *human menopausal gonadotropin*, marketed under the name of Pergonal. Pergonal is a white powder which is dissolved in a salt solution and injected. Though it contains both FSH and LH, frequently additional LH stimulus is given in the form of injections of *HCG* or *human chorionic gonadotropin*. HCG is also a white powder that is dissolved in a salt solution and injected. If there are thyroid problems then the patient may get one of the various forms of thyroid hormones to replace those that are missing. Similarly, your doctor can supplement adrenal glands that are not functioning up to normal levels by administering corticosteroids by mouth. The basic concept of returning to the body what the body is not producing is adhered to.

Thyroid or corticosteroid medication should only be given after laboratory tests show deficient gland function. In the past, these drugs had been given even in the face of a normally functioning adrenal or thyroid. The benefit of giving thyroid or corticosteroid medication to anyone with a normal thyroid or adrenal gland must be questioned.

A great deal of attention has been given to and frustration has been engendered by the man who has a poor sperm count but a normal physical examination and laboratory studies. One of the older forms of treatment is the use of corticosteroids or thyroid medication, although there has been little or no success demonstrated with the use of such medication in the presence of normal endocrine functioning. The use of testosterone to suppress sperm production in the hope that, when the medication is stopped, sperm production will rebound to higher levels, has also been tried. This form of therapy is known as *testosterone rebound therapy*, and it too has been questioned in recent years. Indeed, its potential for harm by permanently suppressing sperm count is a hazard. Recently, various regimens using clomiphene, human chorionic gonadotropin (HCG), and/or Pergonal (HMG), have been tried. Though the use of these drugs must be considered experimental at this point, their potential for success in selected cases of the so-called normal infertile males is very promising.

Corrective Surgery

Microsurgical techniques are now available to correct an obstruction of the vas deferens. A surgeon can excise (cut out) the blocked segment of the vas deferens and anastomose (reconnect) the cut segments under the microscope, thus reestablishing continuity of the pathway for sperm release. Using these microsurgical techniques, approximately 60–80 percent of men will produce viable sperm in their ejaculate. Unfortunately, the pregnancy rate at this time appears to be only 35 percent. This may indicate an effect of male antisperm antibodies produced in sperm collected within the testes during the time the vas deferens was obstructed.

Microsurgical anastomosis of the vas deferens is also currently being used to reverse a vasectomy done for sterilization. The desire for the reversal of sterilization has increased with the increased use of sterilization procedures. Microsurgery is probably the best hope at this point for the return of fertility in those men and women who have undergone these procedures.

FOR THE WOMAN

Replacing Hormones

The woman's basic infertility evaluation begins with a general physical evaluation and general hormonal evaluations. These include screening studies for diabetes, thyroid, adrenal, and liver as well as kidney problems. Many infertility specialists automatically include tests that look for male hormone excess and excessive amounts of a different hormone called *prolactin*. If any abnormal activity of these glands or systems is found, returning function to normal levels is an important first step in treatment. Sometimes such abnormalities are associated with subtle ovulation problems that are corrected when hormone function returns to normal.

Inducing Ovulation

If infertility studies show that the female partner is not ovulating at all or is ovulating very rarely, she should be given drugs to induce regular ovulation. The most common drugs used to produce ovulation are *clomiphene* (marketed under the name Clomid), *human menopausal gonodotropin* (referred to as HMG and marketed as Pergonal), and *human chorionic gonadotropin* (referred to as HCG and marketed as Pregnyl).

Clomiphene was originally discovered when pharmaceutical companies were attempting to chemically construct new estrogens for use in oral contraceptives. One molecule produced had very poor estrogen properties but was accidentally found to induce ovulation in women who previously had not ovulated. This drug was clomiphene citrate. It is sold in the United States under the names of Serophene and Clomid. Clomiphene works by causing the hypothalamus to be stimulated. This, in turn, stimulates the pituitary gland to release more FSH and LH. These hormones act upon the ovary to cause a follicle to ripen and eventually rupture, releasing an egg. The result is ovulation. Clomiphene, a tablet, is usually given in five-day courses. A patient usually takes one or more tablets a day for five days. After several days ovulation occurs.

When a fertility drug is mentioned, many people immediately think of the newspaper stories describing the mixed feelings of an infertile couple who have been treated with a fertility drug and are now blessed with a "litter" of children. The drug referred to in the newspaper articles is usually Pergonal and not clomiphene. Though clomiphene may be associated with a slightly increased incidence of multiple births (twins, etc.), the vast majority of women have one baby and multiple births are usually twins and not triplets, quadruplets, or quintuplets. Clomiphene is safer than Pergonal. It is given by mouth rather than injected. If you take clomiphene, your doctor does not need to monitor you with daily laboratory studies, as is necessary with Pergonal.

Clomiphene's chemical structure is very similar to that of some currently used estrogens. Clomiphene diminishes the effect of estrogens already present in the body, and so it is called an "estrogen blocker" or an "antiestrogen." The drug does this by occupying the sites on cell membranes usually filled by potent estrogens. When clomiphene fills these sites it is as if no estrogen were there, and normal estrogenic effects do not occur. This mechanism acts on the hypothalamus, causing it to stimulate the pituitary. The result is that more FSH and LH are produced and released from the pituitary. These hormones in turn stimulate the ovary and follicular development and ovulation follows.

The production of a large quantity of watery cervical mucus at ovulation depends on estrogenic stimulation. When clomiphene is used, occasionally the estrogenic stimulus for this cervical mucus production is diminished, resulting in very little cervical mucus production. With a small amount of cervical mucus production, it becomes difficult for the sperm to enter the uterus and find their way up to the tube and the egg. The result is a paradox. A woman who is not ovulating but has been able to produce cervical mucus, is given clomiphene so that she will make and release eggs on a regular basis. She will ovulate every cycle, but now may not become pregnant because she is producing a small amount of thick cervical mucus. One problem has been replaced by another. It is important for the physician to do a postcoital test so that cervical mucus and the ability of sperm to survive in the mucus can be examined after the appropriate dose of clomiphene has been determined. If cervical mucus production is reduced following clomiphene therapy, a small amount of estrogen can be given at the same time to improve mucus quality and volume and to facilitate pregnancy.

Clomiphene is also used to treat patients who have problems other than anovulation (nonovulation). In some cases a woman may ovulate very irregularly. If it is important that the time of ovulation be known to plan sexual activity more easily or to perform special procedures—such as artificial insemination (to be discussed later in this chapter)—then clomiphene may be administered. Clomiphene can be used to make an irregularly ovulating woman ovulate more regularly and at known times. The fertile period can be known in advance and if the couple's schedules are complex, their personal lives can be arranged so that they can be sure of making love during the woman's most fertile days.

Most women who take clomiphene for anovulation get progressively increasing doses of the drug until a level is reached that produces an apparently normal ovulation. One or more of the following methods determine that normal ovulation has occurred. The patient is asked to take her basal body temperature readings. Then patient and physician look for the classic, biphasic basal body temperature curve usually associated with normal ovulation. The basal body temperature curve is a rather crude test. Some women who ovulate normally are incapable of generating a classical biphasic curve. If it shows ovulation and other tests concur, then the basal body temperature curve may be thought of as supporting evidence that ovulation did result from treatment. If the basal body temperature curve does not show ovulation but other tests are consistent with ovulation, the temperature curve should be ignored. The other tests are plasma progesterone levels drawn at approximately the midportion of the second half of the cycle, and/or an endometrial biopsy. The plasma progesterone level should show elevation of plasma progesterone to levels usually found with normal ovulation. If ovulation has indeed occurred, then an endometrial biopsy should show a secretory endometrium. The usual maximum dose of clomiphene is five tablets a day for five days. There are several different regimens involving clomiphene use and the maximum dose may vary from physician to physician.

If clomiphene therapy is successful, the woman will ovulate in the cycle during which she takes the drug. Since the drug is essentially out of the body within days of its last dose its effect is not felt beyond the cycle in which it is administered. If pregnancy does not occur, clomiphene must be given monthly to maintain regular ovulation. Clomiphene is used to induce ovulation in a woman who wishes to become pregnant, not to produce regular menstrual cycles in a woman who does not. For the latter situation other drugs can be used. As with any medication, care must be taken not to give clomiphene to a pregnant woman for fear of possibly affecting the fetus.

If ovulation does not occur with the maximum dose of clomiphene, then a cycle at the same dose, with an injection of a hormone called human chorionic gonadotropin (HCG) at cycle day fourteen, is added. A certain percentage of patients will ovulate following the HCG injection who did not ovulate on clomiphene alone.

Approximately 80 percent of the women treated with clomiphene will then ovulate. Of those 80 percent, approximately 40–50 percent will become pregnant in a six-month course of treatment. Of those women who do not become pregnant, an additional percentage may respond to clomiphene plus HCG. Approximately 15 percent of the women who do not ovulate are now left. They should consider HMG (Pergonal) and HCG therapy.

This 15 percent represents that group of women whose pituitary gland fails to produce increased amounts of FSH and LH in response to clomiphene. The physician has tried stimulating the hypothalamus to make the pituitary produce more FSH and LH in an effort to produce the maturation of the follicle and the release of an egg from an ovary. Since the pituitary has been unable to do this an obvious solution is to take FSH and LH from another source and give it to the patient, thereby completely bypassing the pituitary as a source of ovarian stimulation. This is precisely what is done with the administration of HMG (Pergonal).

HMG (Pergonal) is an injectable drug that represents crystallized, purified extract of FSH and LH obtained from the urine of menopausal women. Women in their early menopause produce large amounts of FSH and LH excreted in the urine. It was suggested years ago that an economically feasible way of collecting FSH and LH would be to extract and purify these hormones from menopausal urine which is rich in FSH and LH. This is precisely what has been done. The doctor dissolves the crystalline substance in a small amount of fluid and injects the patient with it to stimulate her ovaries to respond. Since these hormones are being administered exogeneously (from a source outside the body), the control of follicular development is less precise than under normal circumstances. The result is that approximately 20 percent of pregnancies resulting from HMG therapy are multiple births. If your doctor is giving you HMG, he or she should carefully monitor you for clinical response and should use laboratory studies to follow estrogen production. With monitoring, the incidence of multiple births has been reduced as has the incidence of overstimulation of the ovary. Overstimulation of the ovaries is a complex clinical picture, known as *hyperstimulation syndrome*, which results in the ovaries growing from their usual olive size to the size of oranges, grapefruit, or larger. If your ovaries become too large, you must be hospitalized and observed for several days or weeks. The use of HMG must be taken quite seriously and requires both the art and the science of medicine.

There are some women who respond to clomiphene by producing a small amount of FSH and LH but not enough to stimulate the ovary to ovulate. These women need not go to treatment with HMG alone, but can benefit by treatment with clomiphene, HMG, and HCG. In these cases the doctor must decide whether to use clomiphene alone, clomiphene and HMG and HCG, or HMG and HCG. Over 95 percent of the women treated with HMG will ovulate. Approximately 50 percent will become pregnant. Not all of the women who ovulate become pregnant because frequently there is more than one problem and inducing ovulation does not correct other causes of infertility.

A new drug, available in the United Kingdom, Canada, Europe, and the United States, is *bromocryptine*. It induces ovulation in some women who may not respond to clomiphene. Bromocryptine is used to treat women who have elevated blood levels of a hormone called prolactin. These women do not menstruate and have breast discharge. In a recent study, this drug has been found to be useful in treating women who are simply anovulatory. A complete discussion of bromocryptine is beyond the scope of this book. At this point I just want to mention the existence of this new medication, that it can be given by mouth rather than injection, and that it holds great promise for the near future in treating infertile anovulatory women.

If your infertility is a result of a hormonal imbalance, whether of thyroid, adrenal, or hypothalamic-pituitary origin, you usually ovulate very few times or not at all during the course of a year. Ovulation can usually be restored by treating the hormonal problem directly, substituting the missing body substances.

I have so far discussed women who are anovulatory, that is, those who do not ovulate. There is another, more subtle form of ovulation problem. Women who do not ovulate do not produce a corpus luteum and therefore do not produce progesterone. Women who do ovulate release an egg from their ovary and then the corpus luteum in the ovary produces progesterone for fourteen days. If pregnancy does not occur, progesterone production stops, and the woman gets her period. Some women ovulate but produce too little progesterone.

Progesterone is produced in the ovary after ovulation by a structure called the corpus luteum. The corpus luteum can be thought of as a progesterone-producing factory; it is also the structure left over from the follicle after the egg is released. The follicle produces the cells that are later used by the corpus luteum to generate progesterone. Progesterone readies the lining of the uterus for implantation and nourishment of the fertilized egg. When too little progesterone is made, it is thought to be the result of poor functioning of the corpus luteum cells. Since these cells come from the follicle, there are some researchers who feel that the defect lies not in the corpus luteum itself but in the follicle.

There are two ways of treating progesterone deficiencies. One is to stimulate the follicle, producing a larger, more ripened follicle and presumably a better corpus luteum following ovulation. Clomiphene and/or HMG can be used to accomplish this. The rationale behind this treatment is to stimulate the body to produce more of its own progesterone. Some ovaries are not capable of responding to such stimulation, so another approach must be found. That approach is called substitution therapy, where progesterone is provided to the body from an outside source. If the body cannot make progesterone, it is given to the woman from the outside.

Both clomiphene and Pergonal can be used to stimulate progesterone production. Because clomiphene is less expensive, can be administered by tablet instead of injection, and has less risk of causing ovarian enlargement and multiple births, your doctor will probably try it before Pergonal. If clomiphene treatment is unsuccessful or results in cervical mucus that is too thick to allow sperm survival even after additional therapy, then your doctor may consider giving you Pergonal or progesterone substitution therapy.

Pergonal, if administered with appropriate monitoring—as described in the section on anovulation—can be quite successful. The risks and benefits are precisely the same as when this drug is used to treat women who do not ovulate.

A different approach is to provide progesterone from outside the body. Natural progesterone cannot be given by mouth; it can only be introduced into the body by injections or suppositories. The suppositories are soft bulletlike structures that are inserted into either the rectum or vagina and allow to melt; they permit the progesterone to be absorbed through the thin skin surrounding the suppository. The effect is that the progesterone is introduced into the body in a manner similar to an injection.

Progesterone can also be given by injection. It is usually supplied in sesame oil and administered by daily intramuscular injections. Some women find these injections unusually painful, so vaginal or rectal suppositories are usually preferred. However, some women will not absorb progesterone efficiently from a suppository; for them, the injectable form is the better choice.

Clomiphene and Pergonal are each administered in the first portion of the cycle because it is their function to stimulate the development of the follicles. The better the development of the follicle, the better the corpus luteum development, and the more progesterone produced. Progesterone is administered in the second half of the cycle following ovulation. At the time of the expected period a pregnancy test is performed. If it is negative the progesterone is stopped for that cycle. The pregnancy test is required because some women will become pregnant and yet have vaginal bleeding at the time of the expected period. If the progesterone is stopped at this point, the pregnancy will usually not continue. It is important that you have documentation that you are not pregnant before stopping the progesterone.

If you are pregnant, it is important to continue daily progesterone doses until approximately the tenth week of pregnancy. Progesterone is needed to ready the lining of the uterus to support and nourish the early embryo. But you will be taking a drug during a time when the organs of the fetus are being formed. Whenever possible, you should not take any medication during pregnancy. On the other hand, if you stop taking progesterone, the pregnancy may not continue. There are some studies that seem to show there may be an increased risk of fetal abnormality if progesterone is taken during pregnancy. There are other studies—larger and more statistically significant—that appear to show that there is little if any increased risk of fetal abnormality in offspring exposed to progesterone while still in their mother's uterus. The risk of fetal abnormality associated with progesterone exposure appears to be little, if any, but we can never be sure. It is reassuring, however, to know that progesterone has been used for more than thirty years and so if some delayed fetal defect were to occur, such as has been seen with DES, researchers would have had enough opportunity to see it.

It is important to understand that the progesterone discussed above is natural, not synthetic. There are certain drugs that are derivatives of other hormones, such as testosterone, that have been changed in structure to act like progesterone. These drugs have been created because they can be administered in tablet form and will have many of the same biological effects as progesterone. However, these substances, known as progestins or progestogens, are associated with fetal abnormalities if given during pregnancy.

Treatment usually first involves either clomiphene or Pergonal because if they do correct the progesterone deficiency, there is no need for a drug to be continued in early pregnancy. If these drugs are not successful in correcting the progesterone deficiency or they do not lead to pregnancy, then your doctor may have you take progesterone.

The best way of determining whether or not the medication has corrected a progesterone deficiency is to do a pretreatment endometrial biopsy and then repeat the biopsy during a treatment cycle. If the lining of the uterus shows proper development and no progesterone deficiency during a treatment cycle, then the therapy would probably be associated with a high probability of pregnancy. If you cannot tolerate an endometrial biopsy, then your doctor can take a blood progesterone level approximately one week after ovulation. There are some women who have had normal blood progesterone levels but will have a poorly developing uterine lining. A normal blood progesterone level may lull both patient and physician into a false sense of security. As some women find the endometrial biopsy very painful, and since some evaluation is better than none at all, for these women a test of blood progesterone level is an acceptable second choice.

Structural Problems

There is no medicine that will correct a structural abnormality such as an abnormally shaped uterus or closed Fallopian tubes. The only solution is surgery. A doctor usually diagnoses structural abnormality with a hysterosalpingogram and confirms it by endoscopy, be it hysteroscopy, culdoscopy, or laparoscopy. Once the problem has been defined, you and your doctor must consider surgery.

In a woman, the structural abnormalities may be associated with the vagina, the cervix, the uterus, or the Fallopian tubes. It is possible for the woman to have a long wall, running lengthwise down the vagina, acting as a partial obstruction to proper intercourse. Or the vagina may be partially obstructed by a wall extending from side to side. This may be an unusually thick hymen or a wall further within the vagina that effectively seals off the route through which sperm would enter the cervix. In each case the surgical solution is fairly simple. The wall (septum) is surgically removed and the continuity of the vagina is restored.

The cavity of the uterus may have some structures distorting its cavity, projecting into it or somehow affecting its surface area. This may be a result of a fibroid, technically known as a myoma, or a septum (wall), projecting into the uterine cavity. A fibroid is a benign tumor found in approximately 20 percent of all women. In many cases it may be present in various sizes and have absolutely no reproductive significance. However, if the mass is in such a position as to distort the uterine cavity or to partially close off one or both of the Fallopian tubes, surgical treatment should be considered. The fibroid may cause infertility by preventing pregnancy, or by causing recurrent miscarriages (habitual abortions). In the last case, you become pregnant but the growing embryo impinges upon the fibroid, which causes death of the embryo.

The doctor diagnoses the presence of a fibroid by hysterosalpingogram, by ultrasound, and/or by hysteroscopy. Its treatment involves abdominal surgery with the surgical removal of the tumor. The operation is called a *myomectomy*. (See Figure 6.1.)

If, prior to birth, the parts forming the uterus did not properly grow together, then a woman is born with a wall, either complete or incomplete, within the uterine cavity. The presence of a septum within the uterine cavity may result in infertility or more often, repeated miscarriages. The only treatment is surgical.

The most common approach is abdominal surgery. The surgeon opens the uterus and cuts out the wall. The surgeon then sutures the wall closed and completes the abdominal surgery in the usual way. In about 70 percent of the cases a woman who has had this surgery is able to conceive and carry on uneventfully.

Since this surgery produces a scar in the uterine wall which may represent a potential weakened area, most obstetricians are reluctant to allow such a uterus to be subjected to the stresses of labor. For this reason most women who have had uterine surgery producing a uterine scar, whether performed for the removal of a fibroid or the excision of a septum, are delivered by cesarean section. (See Figure 6.2.)

Fallopian tube reconstructive surgery involves a surgical at-

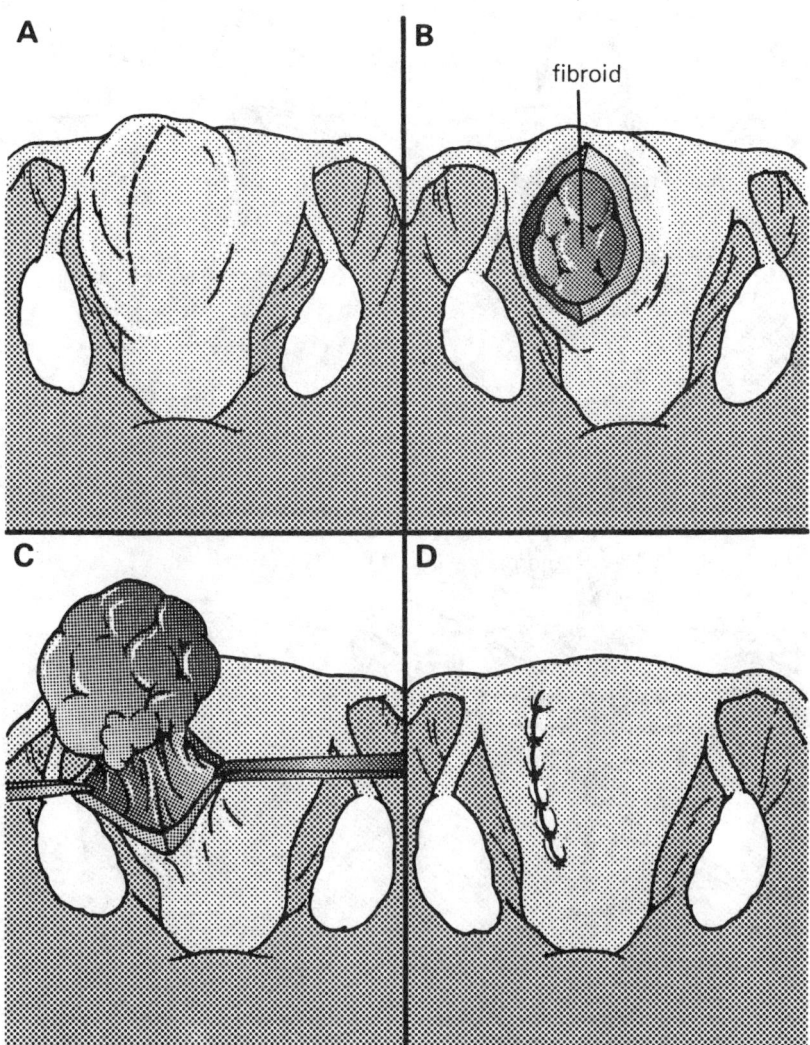

Figure 6.1 *Myomectomy. When it is appropriate, a fibroid may be surgically removed from the uterus and the defect closed.*

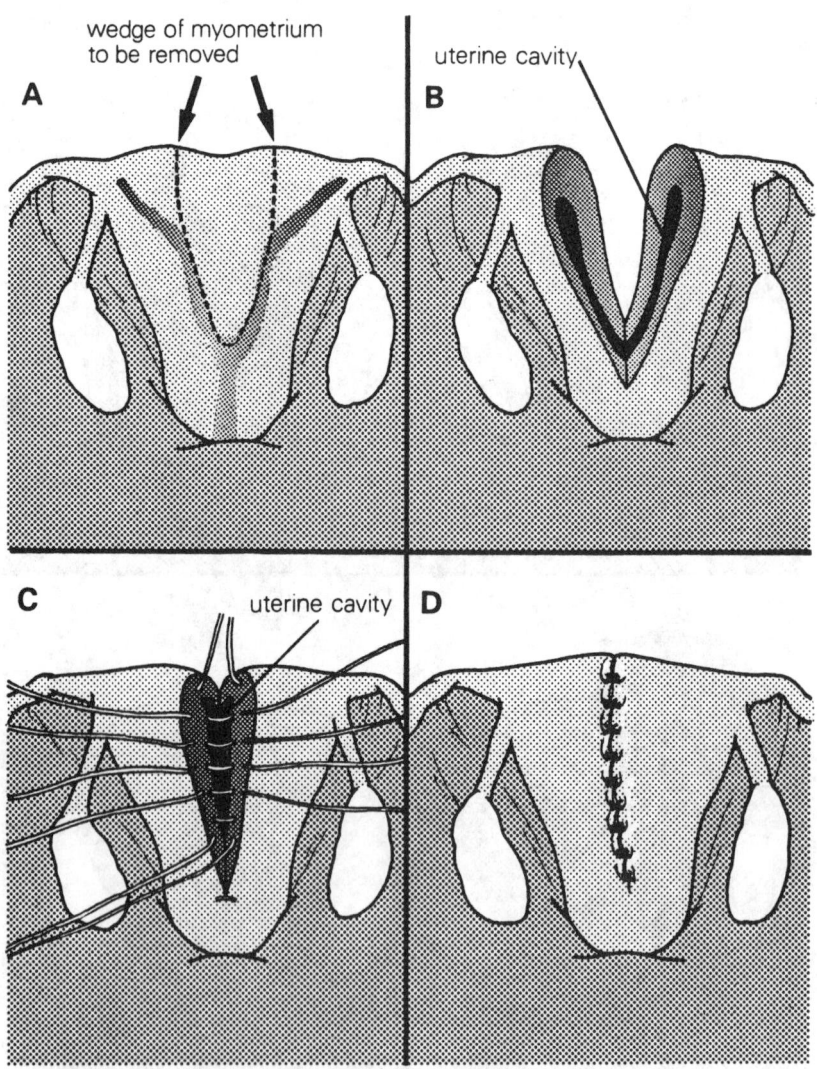

Figure 6.2 *The removal of a septum from a uterus.*
A. *The uterus containing the septum.*
B. *Cutting out the septum.*
C. *Sewing the uterus closed.*
D. *The reconstructed uterus.*

tempt to restore the anatomy of a Fallopian tube. The Fallopian tube is a muscular, movable tubal structure which at one end is connected to the uterus and at the other end forms a funnel-like structure called the fimbria. The outer surface of the Fallopian tube is covered with a slippery membrane called the *peritoneum*. The inner channel of the Fallopian tube is covered with a multifolded lining with many tiny moving hairlike projections called the cilia. This lining, the *endosalpinx*, produces a fluid secretion. The contraction of the muscular layer of the tube, the beating of the hairlike cilia, and the movement of the fluid all combine to move the sperm and the egg through the Fallopian tube.

If scar tissue forms around the outside surface of the tube, the movement of this tube and the ability of the fimbria to pick up an egg are drastically reduced. The surgical solution for this is to cut away the scar tissue, allowing free movement of the tube. If all structures are normal after the surgical procedure and if the Fallopian tube is left totally undamaged, then the probability of becoming pregnant and achieving delivery is quite good, on the order of 70–80 percent.

The procedure, called *lysis of adhesions*, may be done by using laparoscopy. Laparoscopy involves inserting a telescopelike device through the navel and viewing the abdominal contents. If the surgeon finds the tubes are covered with very thin weblike adhesive bands, the surgeon can insert an additional instrument to cut away and break up these bands. If the bands of connective tissue are more dense, using laparoscopy or culdoscopy becomes dangerous. Instead, the surgeon can make a lower abdominal incision and enter the abdomen as for regular surgery. Then the surgeon cuts the scar tissue bands away and closes the abdomen. (See Figures 6.3 and 6.4.)

An obstruction that blocks the channel of the tube, can only be corrected by surgically *excising* (cutting away) that obstructed segment of the tube that is blocked and then *anastomosing* (rejoining) the healthy tube segments. Removing a portion of tube and then rejoining the remaining portions is called *excision and anastomosis*. This is probably one of the most exciting and promising areas of infertility surgery at this time. Recent advances in microsurgery—using very fine suture and a

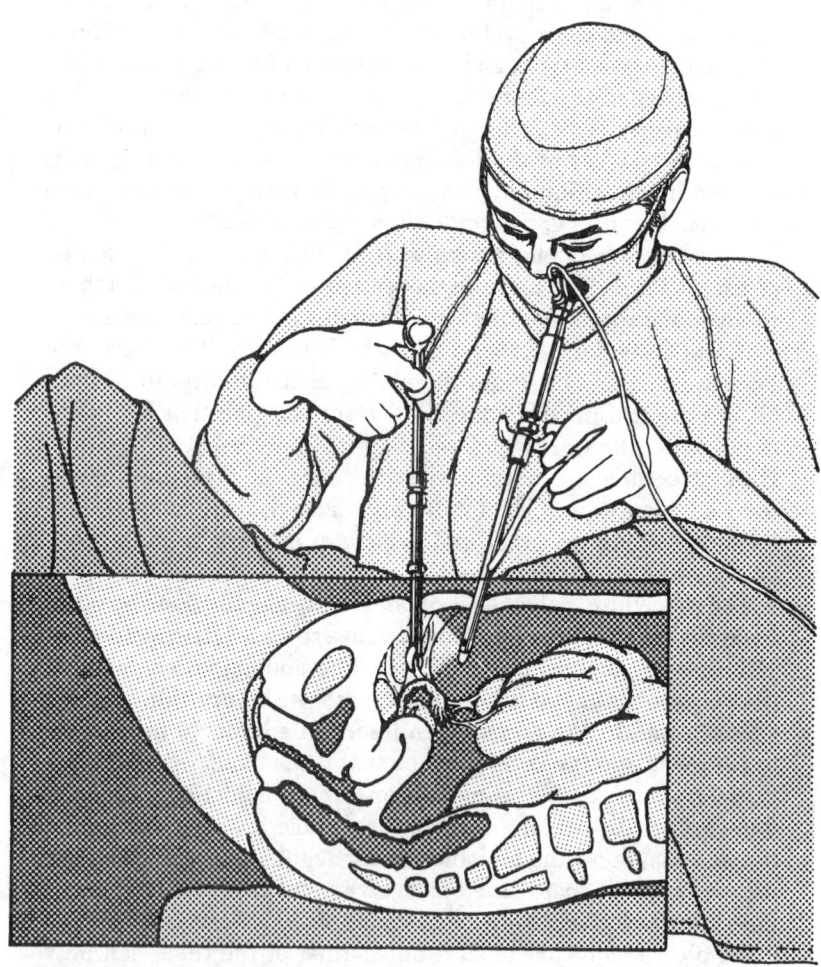

Figure 6.3 *Cutting adhesions with laparoscopic instrument and under laparoscopic observation.*

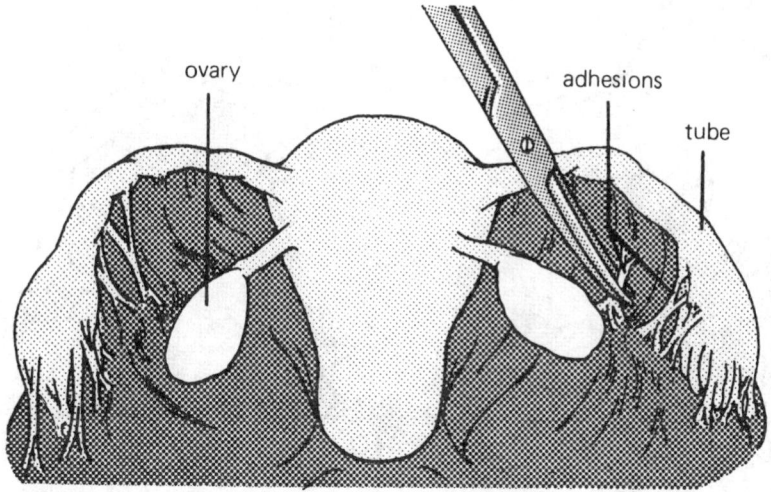

ovary   adhesions

tube

Figure 6.4 *Adhesions being cut away.*

microscope—have significantly improved the results of such surgery. Microsurgery results in almost twice as many live births as regular tubal surgery. The live birthrate using microsurgery to reverse tubal ligation—a sterilization procedure—in selected cases is approximately 75 percent. The live birthrate using conventional surgery is approximately 30 percent. (See Figure 6.5.)

If an obstruction is at the middle of the Fallopian tube, the surgeon can cut away the obstructed area and rejoin the tube using microsurgery. If the obstruction is at the junction of the Fallopian tube and the uterus, the surgeon can cut away the obstruction here too and use microsurgical technique to rejoin the tube to the surface of the uterus. If the obstruction is within the wall of the uterus at the point where the tube enters the uterus, then the surgeon must reimplant the Fallopian tube into the uterine wall. Each of these procedures is associated with its own success rate, depending on the surgical techniques and the amount of damage done to the Fallopian tube.

The most significant lesion in the Fallopian tube is an obstruc-

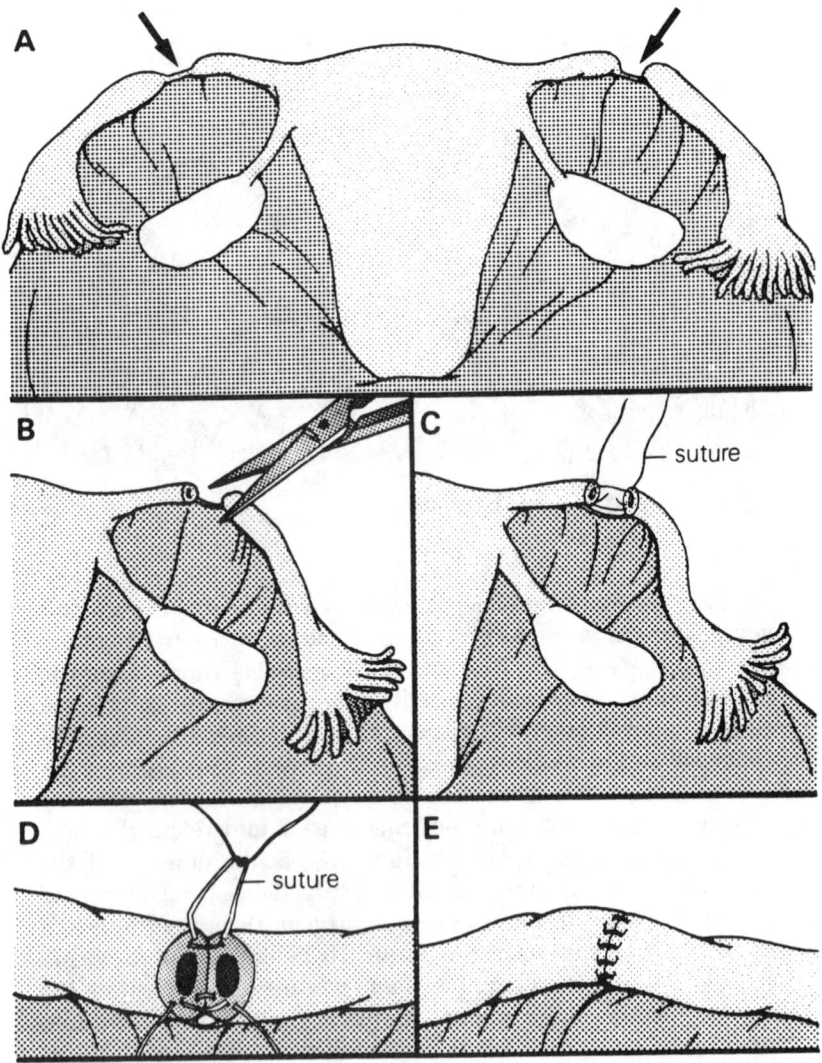

Figure 6.5 *Reversing a tubal ligation. The obstructed segment of each tube is cut out and the tube segments sewn back together (anastomosis).*

tion to the fimbria. A chronic inflammation can cause the fimbria—the funnel-shaped structure at the end of the tube—to become stuck together. The tube becomes enlarged, forming essentially a bag of fluid. The lining of the tube may become irreversibly damaged. The folds of this tissue and the hairlike cilia may be permanently destroyed. The muscles within the Fallopian tube may be destroyed and scar tissue will grow in its place. The result is that all the structures needed to allow an egg to be picked up and moved along the tube are destroyed. A severely scarred midportion of the tube may be removed and the tube rejoined, but if the end of the tube is scarred there is no way of substituting for it. As of today, in spite of a great deal of work, there is no artificial device that can be used to replace the fimbria or the entire Fallopian tube. The blunted sacklike end of the tube may be opened by one of a variety of surgical procedures and sutured in an open position. Occasionally, some regeneration (regrowth) of the lining tissue may occur, and pregnancy does follow. The pregnancy rate following such fimbrial surgery, known as *salpingostomy,* is approximately 15–45 percent. (See Figure 6.6.)

Fallopian tube surgery must not be taken lightly. All surgery is associated with some risk. With Fallopian tube surgery, failure of the surgery does not simply mean that you will not become pregnant. You may become pregnant, but the fertilized egg may be trapped within the Fallopian tube instead of your uterus and the embryo will grow within the tube. This is known as a *tubal pregnancy* and is potentially dangerous because as the embryo grows, the tube may tear and sudden abdominal bleeding occur. The amount and degree of bleeding may be such that you are thrown into sudden shock or may even die. When you and your doctor consider tubal surgery, you must weigh the risks and the benefits carefully. You must balance your extreme desire to bear a child against the risks of tubal pregnancy. Most pregnancies that occur following tubal surgery occur in the uterus and not in the Fallopian tube. As techniques improve, the incidence of tubal pregnancy decreases.

Endometriosis is a condition in which the tissue usually found lining the uterine cavity is also found outside the uterus. Since

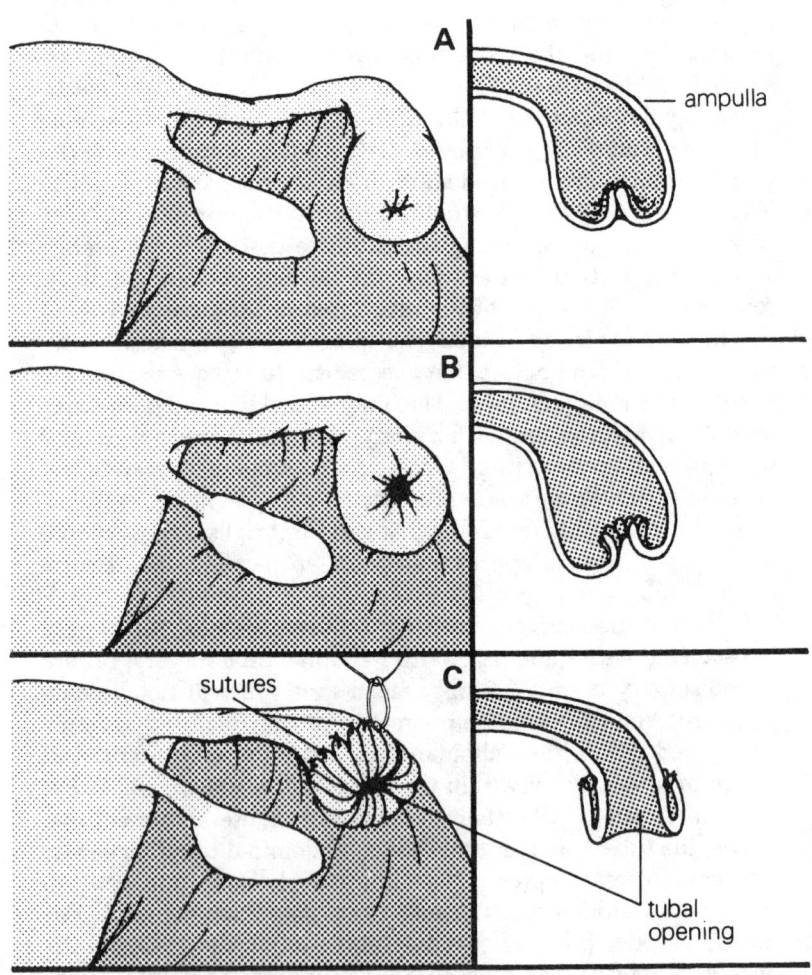

Figure 6.6 *Salpingostomy. A hydrosalpinx may be surgically opened and reconstructed. This procedure is known as a salpingostomy.*
A. *The hydrosalpinx before being opened.*
B. *The clubbed end is carefully opened along the natural folds of the tissue.*
C. *The fimbria are then turned inside out, like the petals of a flower, and sewn into position.*

this material is very irritating to its surrounding tissue, it may cause pain, scarring, and infertility. I reviewed endometriosis as a cause of infertility in Chapter 4. Endometriosis may be treated by drugs and/or by actually cutting away or burning the areas of endometriosis.

Before your doctor begins any treatment, you'll undergo an endoscopy, either culdoscopy or laparoscopy. This procedure allows the physician to directly observe abdominal contents and examine them for endometriosis by means of a telescope inserted into your body. The doctor can confirm the diagnosis of endometriosis and see the extent and amount of scarring the endometriosis has caused.

If there are large ovarian cysts filled with endometriosis, called *endometriomas*, or if there is extensive spread with much scarring, surgery may be the preferred treatment. If there is a small amount of endometriosis, then drug therapy may be used.

Endometriosis depends upon the presence of estrogen for its growth. If the effect of estrogen could be diminished or if the amount of estrogen produced in the patient's body could be reduced temporarily, then the endometriosis would shrivel up. The object of drug treatment is to produce just such a state. This can be accomplished by using Danocrine (danazol), Provera (medroxyprogesterone), or oral contraceptives given in a noncyclic manner. The chosen drug is given daily for about a six-month period, exactly how long may vary depending on the extent of the disease and your response to treatment. The areas of endometriosis shrink to small areas of scar tissue much smaller than their pretreatment size. If the endometriosis was surrounded by scar tissue and adhesions, these scars will remain after the drug treatment and may continue to prevent conception. They can only be treated surgically.

In that case, the surgeon enters the abdomen and removes each area of endometriosis. Then the surgeon closes any openings created and closes the abdomen carefully with fine suture material.

Your doctor may combine the two treatment methods. You may receive a course of drug therapy before surgery to shrink the affected areas and simplify the operation. Or you may have drug treatment after surgery to ensure the complete removal of every trace of endometriosis. In some cases drug therapy alone can offer successful treatment resulting in pregnancy. (See Chapter 9.)

Polycystic ovary syndrome is a particular kind of anovulation in which the ovaries develop many small cysts and become enlarged. In an extreme form known as *Stein-Leventhal syndrome*, affected women become obese and develop a masculinized hair distribution. Polycystic ovary syndrome, referred to as PCO syndrome, can be treated like any form of anovulation. In some cases, after a complete infertility evaluation the woman may be considered for clomiphene therapy. If you do not ovulate, your doctor may give you clomiphene and HCG together. If this is unsuccessful then Pergonal (HMG) and HCG treatment may be used.

If all of these forms of treatment are unsuccessful or if your physician feels that the use of Pergonal is not appropriate for you, then your doctor may consider a surgical procedure called a *wedge resection*. An ovarian wedge resection consists of removing a wedged-shaped segment from each ovary and then sewing the ovary closed. This procedure induces ovulation in women with PCO syndrome by shifting the metabolism of the ovary. Drug treatment using clomiphene is usually tried before surgery because about 80 percent of PCO women treated with drugs will ovulate without surgery. A significant percentage of women who have had wedge resections develop adhesions around their ovaries and tubes. Though they may ovulate after surgery, they may have difficulty becoming pregnant because of these adhesions. (See Figure 6.7.)

ARTIFICIAL INSEMINATION

Artificial insemination is the introduction of sperm into the woman's reproductive tract using a syringe or other device rather than a penis. There are two forms of artificial insemination. A woman may have the sperm of her partner put into her reproductive system or may have the sperm of another man inserted. In the first case, the process is called *artifical insemination—*

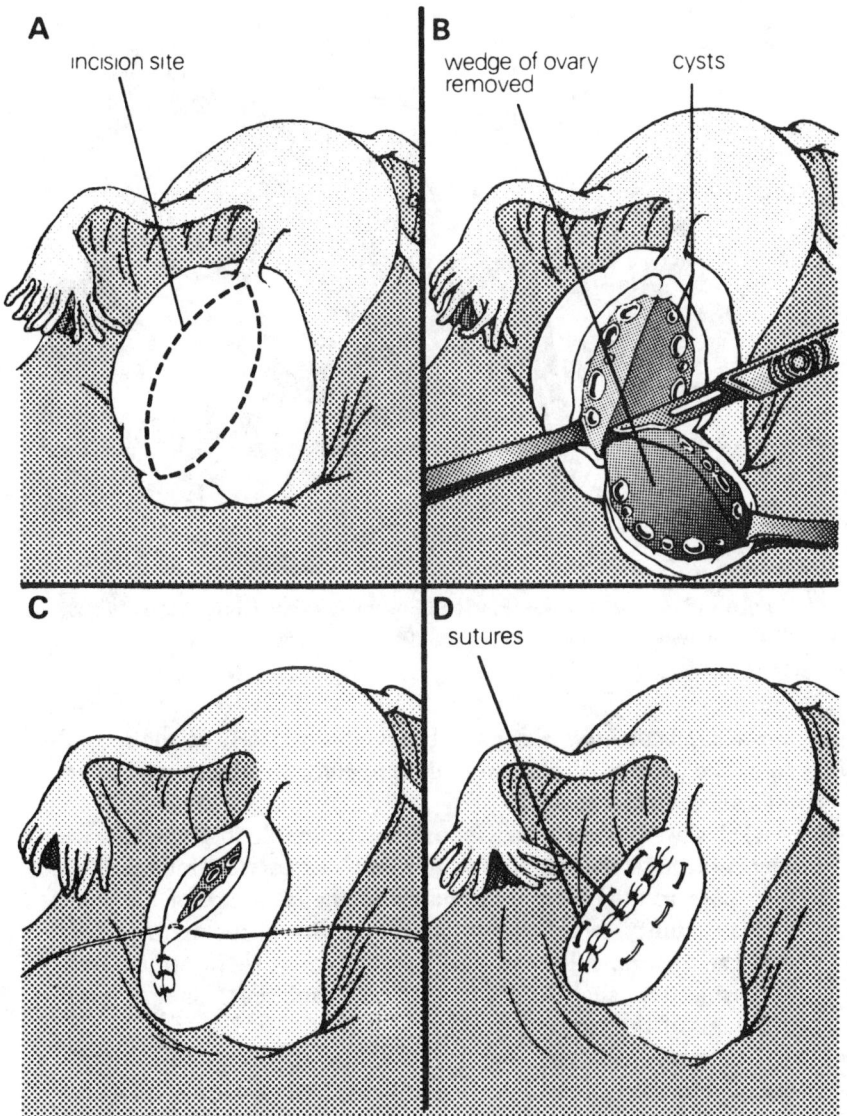

Figure 6.7 *Ovarian wedge resection. A wedge-shaped segment of ovary is removed and the ovary is then sewn closed.*

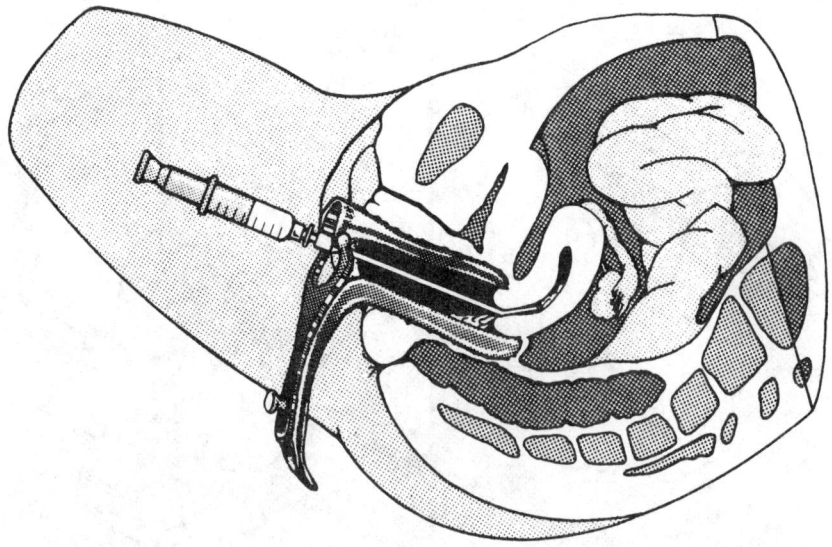

Figure 6.8 *Artificial insemination. Sperm is placed into the cervix or vagina using a syringe and a long tube.*

homologous or *husband,* and abbreviated as AIH. In the second case, the process is referred to as *artificial insemination—donor,* and abbreviated as AID.

AIH is used when a man is technically unable to place his own sperm through the female's vagina into her cervical mucus. This may be a result of an abnormality of the structure of his penis or his inability to achieve sufficient rigidity of his penis to pass into the vagina. AIH can also be used when there are cervical abnormalities, such as local antibody problems, or structural problems of the cervical canal.

The sperm cells used for artificial insemination can be introduced into the woman's cervical mucus, thus allowing the sperm to swim into the reproductive tract in the usual way. Sometimes a sperm sample is of very small volume, or there may be just a borderline number of sperm cells present in the specimen. In order to prevent the sperm cells from being lost in the volume of the vagina, your doctor or a technician can hold the specimen tightly against the cervical mucus with a plastic cervical cap. In this form of artificial insemination, your doctor places the plastic cap over your cervix and injects the sperm sample into the cap through a long plastic tube with a valve on it. Your doctor places the specimen in the cap, closes the valve, and the specimen is held tightly, delivering a greater number of sperm cells into your reproductive tract.

Another variation of artificial insemination can be used if the woman produces very little cervical mucus, or if the quality of the sperm sample used is marginal. Here, instead of delivering the sample into the cervical mucus, your doctor injects it through the cervical canal directly into the uterine cavity. The result is a relatively large number of sperm cells introduced into the uterine cavity. This procedure, known as *intrauterine insemination*, sometimes abbreviated as IUI, would appear to be the way to drastically increase pregnancy rates. But in fact, the probability of pregnancy following intrauterine insemination is not markedly increased over regular insemination. There are certain exceptions to this statement. In cases where cervical mucus production is very poor, either in quality, quantity, or both, or where sperm samples are truly borderline in quality, there can be an increase in pregnancy rate using intrauterine insemination. For use with sperm samples of normal quality and/or good cervical mucus, intrauterine insemination appears to be of little if any benefit.

If the man is sterile and the woman has no reproductive problems, then donor artificial insemination can be used. In this case, sperm is obtained from an unidentified man who is screened to match the characteristics of the male partner of the infertile couple. The sperm is then placed into the reproductive system of the woman.

The sperm used for donor insemination can either be fresh or obtained frozen from a sperm bank. In the case of a fresh specimen, the sperm sample is obtained from a matched donor and is introduced into the woman's reproductive tract by artificial insemination, usually within two to four hours of production.

With banked sperm, the specimen has been preserved, frozen, transported to the doctor's office, and thawed just prior to insemination. In general, pregnancy rates following donor insemination using fresh sperm are slightly higher than using banked sperm. But a good bank that uses carefully screened donors with good quality sperm samples and that stores the specimens under carefully controlled conditions can achieve pregnancy rates not much different than they would have been if fresh specimens had been used. There are certain advantages and disadvantages to each approach. Fresh samples that are produced by donors are associated with higher pregnancy rates but are not always available at the date and time of a woman's appointment for insemination. Bank samples can usually be made more easily available on an as-needed basis.

A more important factor in the selection of a donor for artificial insemination is the possibility of the woman developing Acquired Immunodeficiency Syndrome, or AIDS. AIDS appears to be the result of an infection by a virus. The probable causative agent is known in the United States as Human T-Cell Leukemia virus type III, and abbreviated as HTLV-III or HIV. HIV virus can be spread through seminal fluid and therefore artificial insemination may transmit AIDS to the recipient woman. Thus, it becomes critical to screen any donor who is chosen for artificial insemination to be sure that he does not carry the AIDS virus. Unfortunately, it is very difficult to test for the HIV virus itself.

Once infected by HIV, a person will produce antibodies to that virus. By screening donors for HIV viral antibodies and selecting only those who are HIV negative, we should have a group of people with a low risk of carrying AIDS. However, it appears that it takes at least two months and possibly more than one year, for someone exposed to the AIDS virus to develop antibodies to HIV. In order to know that a specimen is truly free of the AIDS virus, the donor must have had an HIV antibody study that was negative at the time of production and that remained negative three to six months—and even twelve months or more—later. The best way to do this is to use banked sperm. Most banks will have a donor produce a sperm sample, which will be banked at that time. At the same time, a blood sample is drawn and tested for HIV antibodies. If the antibody studies are negative, the specimen is kept in the bank, and the donor is brought back three months later. At that time he is retested for HIV antibodies and if once again he is found to be negative, then it is believed that at the time of production of the original specimen he did not harbor the AIDS virus. Thus, a specimen is released for use in artificial insemination only after it has been banked for three months and the donor has had two negative HIV studies three to twelve months apart.

This sort of screening cannot be done with a fresh specimen used immediately after production. If a donor being tested for HIV antibodies on the day that he produces his specimen is found to be antibody negative, we still cannot be sure that he is not carrying the virus for he may not yet have had the opportunity to produce antibodies. Some donor insemination programs still do use fresh specimens but care must be taken to test the donors frequently. With all of the most precise testing, the greatest safety exists with banked specimens of appropriately screened donors.

Approximately 50 to 70 percent of couples using donor insemination achieve pregnancy. The success rate of artificial insemination using the partner's sperm varies tremendously and depends upon the existence or absence of other factors further compromising a woman's fertility.

VIGOROUS EXERCISE AND FERTILITY

Of the various crazes to spread through the United States, the desire to improve one's physical fitness is probably one of the most reasonable and helpful. Recently both men and women have been exercising extensively—jogging, running, aerobic dancing, and long-distance marathon running. The benefits to the cardiovascular system appear to be beyond dispute, although the projected effects on longevity still remain to be proven. Some discussion revolves around the effect of running on reproductive ability. Like many simply phrased questions, the answer is complex. For most people, running causes a loss of fatty tissue, among other things. In the human female, fatty tissue acts very much like an endocrine gland, converting some of the substances from the adrenal gland to estrogen. An obese woman has a large quantity of fatty tissue and therefore is producing a lot of extra estrogen. In a certain sense, this estrogen acts like a built-in birth control pill. It is perhaps for this reason that a significant percentage of very overweight women tend not to ovulate. If vigorous exercise results in weight loss and a total reduction in fat, then, for these women running may have a very definite benefit. On the other hand, if exercise reduces the percentage of fat below a certain point, ovulation seems to become less likely. An important factor in long-distance running is the creation of the stress situation, causing an increased cardiac rate and exercising the heart muscle over an extended period of time. If running produces an overall stress situation, the result may be lack of ovulation. This lack of ovulation is not a result of the increased load on the heart but may be a symptom of physiological or psychological stress in the central nervous system. Rapid fluctuations in weight, which may very well follow long-distance running, may also produce an anovulatory state.

A woman's menstrual flow itself may be changed with exercise. Studies have shown that running twenty to forty miles per week—or doing other equivalent exercise—is associated with a reduction in the amount of a woman's menstrual flow. Some women athletes will actually cease menstrual bleeding during times of aggressive workouts. It does not seem to make a difference whether a woman is a runner, swimmer, dancer, gymnast, or water polo player. The important factor appears to be the amount and intensity of the aerobic exercise in which she is engaged. The cause of this change in menstrual pattern is unknown. The change in percentage of total body fat occurring with exercise, while appearing to be an important factor, is not the only one. Changing menstrual patterns usually reflect changes in ovulation and progesterone production and may, therefore, be associated with a decreased probability of achieving a pregnancy.

Vigorous exercise may be very helpful to some women and detrimental to others. Although runners have been studied at several institutions, there does not yet seem to be agreement on the percentage of women who stop ovulating after starting a running program as opposed to the percentage who were not ovulating and who began making eggs after starting to run. It does seem clear, however, that there is a small percentage of women who cease ovulating as well as those who continue to ovulate but develop progesterone deficiencies when they undertake a vigorous program of exercise. The mechanism that causes this is not known, but the changes that result do not appear to be permanent. Furthermore, there is no reason to believe at this time that women who stop ovulating after beginning an exercise program will be more difficult to treat than any other women who do not ovulate. Clomiphene or Pergonal seem to work quite successfully. However, since no treatment is always better than even the most benign treatment, I frequently suggest that women who are aggressive exercisers and who have stopped ovulating after beginning their exercise program stop temporarily.

It is important to remember that if a woman who exercises stops ovulating, it is not necessarily the exercise that caused the cessation of ovulation. There may be some other cause, and the woman might have stopped ovulating at the same time even if no exercise program had existed. It is therefore important that we not assume that an ovulation problem is necessarily due to exercise. All women who exercize vigorously should be evaluated just as any woman who has an ovulation problem. In this way, appropriate diagnoses will not be missed.

ORAL CONTRACEPTIVES

With the extensive use of oral contraceptives, it is not uncommon to hear of a woman who apparently does not ovulate and menstruate after stopping use of "the pill." In medical terminology this is called *postpill amenorrhea*. Though it is spoken of frequently, postpill amenorrhea occurs in less than 1 percent of women who have used oral contraceptives. It is not related to how long a woman uses the pill. Women who have used birth control pills for several months have the same incidence of postpill amenorrhea as those who have used the medication for years. And most cases of postpill amenorrhea may have little to do with oral contraceptive use.

Women who have postpill amenorrhea fall into three groups. The first is comprised of those who ovulated infrequently before starting oral contraceptives and continue to be anovulatory after stopping them. In this case the lack of ovulation is the continuation of a previous menstrual pattern rather than a result of having taken birth control pills.

The second group is composed of women who had regular menses prior to birth control pill use but do not ovulate after stopping the pill. It appears that most of these women would have stopped ovulating even if they had not used oral contraceptives. This is demonstrated statistically by noting that the incidence of anovulation and infertility among nonpill users is the same as among those who used oral contraceptives. If birth control pills caused lasting anovulation, there would be more amenorrhea and infertility in the group of ex-pill users. This is *not* the case.

The last group are those women whose ovulatory centers may have remained suppressed after the use of oral contraceptives. The result is the failure to resume normal ovulation after birth control pills have been stopped. This group represents a very small percentage of all postpill amenorrhea patients.

It is very difficult to separate the second from the third group just mentioned. In a sense it is of little significance since members of all three groups can usually be treated equally well and successfully. The therapy for anovulation as discussed earlier in this chapter is used. Most women with postpill amenorrhea respond well to clomiphene treatment.

The Court of Last Resort

When all appropriate forms of treatment for infertility have been used and pregnancy has not resulted, in vitro fertilization should be considered. This procedure, frequently called the "test-tube baby procedure," and some of its variations, such as GIFT, are discussed in detail in Chapter 11.

Various problems each have their own approach and their own degree of success. Anovulation can be treated with medication, inducing ovulation in somewhat more than 95 percent of cases and pregnancy in about 60 percent of those cases. Uterine reconstruction is associated with approximately 80 percent live birthrate. Fallopian tube reconstruction is associated with approximately 15–75 percent live birthrate, depending on the location and degree of damage to the tube.

Not being able to become pregnant is not the only reproductive problem that requires attention. In the next chapter I will discuss miscarriage.

CHAPTER 7

Conception Is Not the Only Problem: Miscarriage

INFERTILITY IS the inability of a couple to produce a pregnancy. But what do we say about couples who conceive, only to miscarry early in pregnancy? Strictly speaking, these people are not infertile because they can conceive. Nonetheless, if the losses are repetitive and not isolated events the result is the same as infertility—they are unable to have children.

Because miscarriage is a separate category from infertility I present it here as a separate chapter. In most cases the diagnostic procedures and the treatments are the same as or similar to those already presented in the diagnosis and treatment of infertility. Where appropriate I will briefly review these techniques here to emphasize their use in the evaluation and treatment of miscarriage.

It is an extremely difficult and upsetting experience for two people who have just celebrated the joy of conception to find that their pregnancy is abruptly over. Their questions are usually, "Why us?" "Why did it happen?" and "Will this happen again?" Let us begin by answering these questions.

It is difficult to tell any individual couple why they lost their pregnancy. However, we can make a certain number of general statements that are still relevant.

The loss of an early pregnancy is not at all unusual. Approximately 15–20 percent of all pregnancies are lost before the twenty-sixth week. In layman's language, such a loss of conception is known as a *miscarriage*. In medical terminology, the loss of a fetus before the twenty-sixth week of pregnancy is an *abortion*. The technical use of "abortion" does not imply that the loss of the pregnancy resulted from manipulation or a surgical procedure as it does in layman's language. An abortion may be induced, meaning that it has resulted from some manipulation, or spontaneous, implying that nothing was done to bring it on. Spontaneous abortion, that is, a miscarriage, is the subject of the discussion in this chapter.

If you become pregnant and have a miscarriage it is very probable that this will be an isolated event. You will probably be able to conceive again, have an uneventful pregnancy, and deliver a perfectly normal child. Most miscarriages are one-time occurrences and, though upsetting, should only temporarily interrupt your reproductive plans. If you go on to have a total of two consecutive miscarriages it is most likely that a definite problem exists and should be investigated. The latter condition, known as *recurrent abortion*, deprives a couple of the ability to have their own children.

Until very recently, three early fetal losses represented the criterion to begin evaluation for miscarriage. Newer studies strongly suggest that women who have had two consecutive miscarriages have a risk of repetitive fetal loss that is very close to those who have had three consecutive miscarriages. As a result, many physicians now recommend beginning medical evaluation for fetal loss after two miscarriages rather than three.

The first twelve weeks of pregnancy, known as the *first trimester*, is the time of greatest risk for miscarriage, since 86 percent occur during this period.

If a conception is spontaneously and completely expelled from the uterus into the vagina leaving no residual pregnancy tissue in the uterine cavity, it is known as a *complete abortion*. If some tissue is passed and the remainder is retained in the uterus, this is referred to as an *incomplete abortion*. A *missed abortion* occurs when the pregnancy dies and all the tissue remains within the uterus.

No treatment is usually required immediately after a verified complete abortion. On the other hand, a woman with an incomplete or missed abortion should have the tissue removed from the uterus. This is usually done by a minor surgical procedure known as a *dilation and curettage* or a *D & C*. In this procedure, the cervix, the opening of the uterus, is stretched and the lining of the uterine cavity is scraped off or curetted. Performing a D & C helps to diminish the chances of heavy vaginal bleeding and subsequent uterine infection.

CAUSES OF MISCARRIAGE

Most miscarriages are random mistakes of nature that usually are not repeated. It is only when a woman has had two consecutive spontaneous abortions that she should consider a complete medical evaluation. After one miscarriage, the most likely explanation is that of a *blighted ovum* or *blighted pregnancy*. In this instance there is something grossly abnormal about the cells produced from the initial division of the fertilized egg. This may be a result of a defective egg or sperm cell. In a kind of protective mechanism built into most animals, these grossly abnormal masses of cells rarely survive. It is a way of preventing the birth of markedly abnormal offspring. Many of these blighted pregnancies are lost so early that the patient may not even realize that she was pregnant. It is only by careful examination of the menstrual tissue that abnormal products of conception may be found. This condition is probably more common than is believed but is usually not a cause of repetitive miscarriage. A blighted pregnancy is a result of a chance abnormality in the development of an egg or a sperm. In this case, both members of the couple are capable of producing normal cells in the vast majority of cases and these mistakes of nature can occur in anyone without affecting further reproduction.

In the Case of Habitual Abortion

If a woman loses two consecutive pregnancies she is said to have *recurrent abortions*. If she has three or more consecutive miscarriages she is said to have *habitual abortions*. In either case she and her partner can achieve conception and are therefore not strictly infertile. However, their efforts cannot produce a living child. The problem may be related to genetic abnormality, hormonal problems, a uterine abnormality, cervical abnormality, or infection.

Some men and women may carry an abnormal genetic information in their chromosomes. This defective hereditary material may not express itself in that particular individual but it combines with the genetic material from the partner to form a pregnancy that cannot live. Certain genetic combinations and abnormalities will not allow a pregnancy to continue. If a couple produce pregnancies which end in miscarriages, particularly within the first twelve weeks of pregnancy, the doctor must seriously consider a *genetic abnormality*. In this case, as opposed to the blighted pregnancy situation described above, the couple is producing defective genetic material much of the time and not on rare occasions. Genetic studies, called *karyotyping*, must be done to diagnose such genetic problems and to tell such a couple what the probability is of their ever being able to produce a pregnancy that will survive.

Another cause of habitual abortion is a disturbance in one of the woman's hormonal systems. Since the woman's body provides the environment for the pregnancy, any significant biochemical disturbance of this environment may seriously affect the viability of the fetus. Overfunctioning or underfunctioning of the thyroid gland can lead to a loss of pregnancy. Abnormal functioning of the adrenal gland can also result in a miscarriage. If you are a diabetic whose blood sugars are not under control, the conception may be lost early or at any time right through to the end of pregnancy. Diabetics must be managed very carefully during pregnancy. A progesterone deficiency that is not significant enough to prevent pregnancy may exist and be just severe enough to allow the loss of a new conception. Your doctor can diagnose any of these hormonal abnormalities by taking a blood sample and testing it for the appropriate hormonal products. In screening for diabetes, a glucose tolerance test would be most appropriate.

In the process of development, the fertilized egg implants on the lining of the uterine cavity and then progressively enlarges in size. The embryo depends upon the blood supply in the uterine wall below the area of implantation for its nourishment and on the uterine cavity for a protected space into which it can grow. If the blood supply to the developing embryo is diminished or if because of abnormalities in the structure of the uterine wall it must compete for growing space in the uterus, then a miscarriage may result.

The uterus may contain a noncancerous tumor known as a myoma or fibroid. Such a tumor may be entirely within the uterine wall or may project into the uterine cavity. If the fertilized egg implants on the tumor, the tissue is not capable of supplying a sufficient blood supply to sustain its growth. Furthermore, as the conception grows, so will the fibroid. Often the tumor will compress the uterine cavity providing insufficient room for the growing pregnancy. By impairing the blood supply and/or reducing the uterine cavity space, the fibroid is capable of producing a miscarriage. The presence of such a tumor does not necessarily mean that it is the cause of the abortions. It is possible for the fibroid to be on the outside surface of the uterus without affecting the pregnancy. The uterus must be studied by one of the techniques mentioned below to determine if the fibroid is related to the miscarriages.

Occasionally a woman will have a uterus that appears perfectly normal on the outside but has a wall projecting into the cavity on the inside. Such a wall is known as a *uterine septum* and can act just as a fibroid to produce miscarriages.

The diagnosis of any abnormality of the uterine cavity is usually begun by performing an X-ray called a *hysterosalpingogram*. The uterus, which is made of soft tissue, will not show up on X-ray. However, if the cavity is filled with a fluid that can be seen on X-ray, a photograph of a silhouette of the uterine cavity can be made. Any change of the usual triangular shape of the space may be a result of compression by a fibroid or a uterine septum.

The surface of the uterine cavity can be viewed directly by placing a telescopelike device, called a hysteroscope, through the vagina and cervix into the uterus. This way the fibroid or septum can actually be seen rather than relying on a photograph of a silhouette as with an X-ray. Both of these techniques are discussed in greater detail in Chapter 5.

As the fetus grows, it exerts increasing pressure on the cervix. Circular muscle and connective tissue fibers present within the body of the cervix keep it closed and keep the fetus within the uterine cavity. If these tissue fibers are defective, then the cervix is unable to maintain its closed state against the downward pressure of the uterine contents. When this happens, the cervix opens and the fetus is passed out into the vagina and the outer world, well before it is capable of surviving on its own. This condition is known as an *incompetent cervical os*. Previous miscarriage can make your physician suspect you have an incompetent os. Women with this problem classically describe the painless loss of the fetus as opposed to experiencing the cramps of labor usually felt with other forms of miscarriage. Your doctor can verify the diagnosis by performing a dilation and curettage and actually feeling the kind of resistance the cervical tissue offers to touch.

Mycoplasma, an organism between a virus and a bacteria, has been cited by some as being a cause of habitual abortion. This is still controversial and I only mention it here for the sake of completeness; in the future more definitive work may be done.

Possible Immunological Causes

Some researchers explain that the repetitive loss of pregnancies occurs because the woman's immune system is not working properly. This impressive mechanism recognizes cells that are foreign to the body and distinguishes them from cells that belong to it. The foreign cells are catalogued by the surface structure of the outer coat of their cells and are attacked by substances called *antibodies*. These antibodies and cells that travel with them are very specific to the invading foreign cells. A developing early pregnancy has the genetic composition of both the mother and the father and is therefore distinct and foreign in cell type from that of the mother in which it is developing. Scientists have always been fascinated by the fact that a developing embryo can grow within the uterus of a mother without being attacked by the mother's immunological system. It appears that this wondrous event can occur because the mother's body produces a very special group of substances called *blocking antibodies*. These blocking antibodies prevent the mother's body from recognizing the developing embryo as a foreign agent, and therefore the attacking substances are never produced.

Some researchers feel that a small percentage of miscarriages are caused by the malfunctioning of this blocking antibody system. Just as people's blood cells can be described as being type A, B, O, Rh positive, and Rh negative, so all body cells can be typed by a system called the *HLA system*. When the man and woman producing a pregnancy have HLA tissue types that are very close, these researchers theorize that the embryo that has been produced is not different enough in cell type to produce a blocking antibody in the mother. The embryo may still be different enough to be recognized as foreign by her body defense system, so antibodies specific to the embryo are made and the embryo is destroyed. Researchers who hold this theory have demonstrated—at least in some couples who have had repetitive miscarriages—that the HLA typing indeed can be quite similar between the man and the woman. In some cases, a preparation of the man's white blood cells has been used to inoculate the woman to help stimulate proper blocking antibody production. When the treated couples again attempted pregnancy, the ensuing embryos did not die, and a miscarriage did not result. These researchers have demonstrated that, at least in some people, miscarriage can be associated with HLA similarities between the man and the woman and ensuing miscarriages appear to be prevented by inoculating the woman with the special preparation of white cells from the man.

This therapy is still controversial and should be reserved for special cases where no other causes of recurrent fetal loss have been found.

Connective Tissue Diseases

Another possible cause of recurrent fetal loss is *connective tissue diseases*. Most people are unaware of these disorders. They are problems associated with the substances that hold the cells of our bodies together and include connective tissue diseases, certain types of arthritis, and diseases such as scleraderma. While some of these disorders may have dramatic clinical signs, there are many people who have absolutely no symptoms but whose blood shows changes similar to those seen with connective tissue diseases. The last category is described as people with subclinical forms of the disease.

When women who have had repeated miscarriages are studied for connective tissue diseases, a small percentage will have positive laboratory studies. Women who have connective tissue diseases may have a probability of pregnancy survival that is as low as 6–8 percent. When the connective tissue disease is treated, the pregnancy survival rate increases to approximately 80 percent. Early studies seem to show that women with recurrent pregnancy losses and connective tissue problems can be treated easily with baby aspirin or a cortisonelike drug called prednisone. This simple therapy results in an increased probability of not miscarrying again. Indeed, the chances of carrying a pregnancy can increase ten times.

In evaluating your blood for connective tissue diseases your doctor can test for antinuclear antibodies (ANA) and anticardiolipin (ACA), prothrombin time (PT), and partial thromboplastin time (PTT). Positive results in any of these areas need to be carefully evaluated and the use of prednisone and aspirin—just as the use of any drugs in pregnancy—must be carefully evaluated for risks and benefits.

Environment

The possible role of occupational environmental hazards in producing miscarriages has become increasingly significant. It is difficult to state in any individual case whether or not the loss of a particular pregnancy was the result of exposure to occupational or environmental pollutants. But there are certain substances that are known to adversely affect pregnancies. The environments of hospital operating rooms, including anesthetic gas such as nitrous oxide, have been associated with miscarriage. Exposure to organic solvents in chemical laboratories and research facilities, as well as to copper, lead, arsenic, and cadmium, has been linked to miscarriages. Halogenic polycyclic hydrocarbons, PVCs, and methomercury are just a few other substances that have been a basis for concern. Many of the chemicals and solvents routinely used by hairdressers and cosmetologists may also adversely affect pregnancies. When in doubt, try to remove as many foreign substances from your environment and cut down on—and if at all possible totally stop—smoking, alcohol use, recreational drug use, and any use of prescription and over-the-counter drugs. Whenever possible, ask yourself, "Do I have to use this substance?" before putting anything into your body during pregnancy. If the answer is not an absolute "yes," then don't use the substance.

WHAT DOES NOT CAUSE MISCARRIAGES

I have not yet covered physical or emotional trauma in the discussion of the causes of miscarriage. It is not uncommon for a woman to miscarry and then feel that it was a result of something that she did. She may feel that she engaged in too much activity, that she worried too much, or that she had too much or too little exercise. She may wonder if that extra-long automobile trip had anything to do with her miscarriage. Most of these things are truly irrelevant. The intrauterine environment is a very safe, self-contained fluid medium that is able to sustain tremendous shock. A normally functioning placenta is able to biochemically maintain the needs of a normal fetus. If the environmental stress of everyday activity is enough to upset the balance of the fetus, then we must consider the basic situation so compromised that survival was almost impossible from the beginning. There is no need for individuals or couples to torture themselves with feelings of guilt because of a pregnancy loss. In most cases there was nothing that they did that produced the miscarriage.

TREATMENT

Now that we have reviewed the causes of miscarriage, let us turn to its treatment. Since a single miscarriage is usually not associated with any further reproductive problems, a full evaluation is usually not carried out. For the same reason no treatment is given.

If you have had habitual abortions and your doctor has diagnosed a hormonal problem, you should have blood tests performed to determine thyroid and progesterone levels and adrenal gland function. You should be given whatever hormones you are deficient in. If you have a thyroid deficiency, thyroid medication should be considered. There are several drugs that may be given. Your physician will select the most appropriate medication. If your adrenal glands are not working up to normal levels, your doctor will select one of the corticosteroid drugs to give you. We have already discussed the use of clomiphene or progesterone for progesterone deficiency. You would never take clomiphene during pregnancy, but your doctor may consider your using it before pregnancy.

If a hysterosalpingogram and/or hysteroscopy reveals an abnormality of the uterine contour such as a fibroid or a uterine septum, these abnormalities should be removed by means of abdominal surgery. Several techniques can be used for the removal of the uterine septum. The procedure is basically that of opening the uterus, cutting out the septum or fibroid, and then sewing the uterine wall back together again. For the removal of a fibroid, an incision is made into the wall of the uterus and the fibroid is extracted. The uterine wall opening is then closed. This procedure is known as a *myomectomy*.

If you have an incompetent cervix—indicated by your medical history and confirmed by having a dilation and curettage—your doctor may perform a *Shirodkar procedure*. In this procedure your doctor places a heavy suture material around the cervix, under the covering mucosal tissue. The suture is tied and acts as a substitute for the defective or missing connective tissue. The suture material actually ties the cervix in a closed, normal position. The Shirodkar procedure may be done either before or just after you become pregnant, around the beginning of the second trimester.

If a T-mycoplasma infection is considered to be a reason for miscarriage, both members of the couple should be treated with an appropriate antibiotic, such as doxycycline.

Genetic Causes

If a genetic abnormality is causing miscarriage, then this too can be addressed. If the man carries a gene that will result in an embryo that will usually die and result in a miscarriage, then donor sperm can be used by artificial insemination. The result should be a pregnancy that progresses well. If the miscarriages result from the woman's genetic information, then a donor egg can be provided through in vitro fertilization and the resulting embryo can be put into the woman's body. These options are very real and will be discussed in great detail in Chapter 11.

Even though a single cause for habitual abortion may be found, the remainder of the studies should still be completed. There is a certain small chance that there may be multiple causes for miscarriages. If treatment is to be successful, all of the problems must be defined and corrected.

Habitual abortion, like other problems in reproductive medicine, is being studied in many centers throughout the world. Many advances are expected in the near future both in diagnosis and treatment.

CHAPTER 8
Ectopic Pregnancy

ONCE A couple who have been unable to achieve a pregnancy hear the magic words, "Congratulations, the pregnancy test is positive!" there is an uncontrolled outpouring of relief and joy. After months or years of trying, the first major hurdle toward realizing the birth of their baby has been passed. Upon achieving a pregnancy, thus accomplishing their major goal, a whole new set of concerns is raised. The next major question that both the physician and couple must address is the location of the embryo. The vast majority of the time the embryo will be found inside the uterine cavity. If this is the case, then, barring miscarriage, (discussed in Chapter 7), the pregnancy should progress well and the delightful moment of the delivery of the couple's child should occur. If the pregnancy occurs outside the uterine cavity, there is a high probability of major complications to the mother. A pregnancy located outside the uterine cavity is called an *ectopic pregnancy*. In order to avoid complications, it becomes important to diagnose and treat an ectopic pregnancy as soon as possible. (See Figure 8.1a and 8.1b.)

AN OVERVIEW

In order for a pregnancy to take place, an egg is released by the ovary and picked up by the fimbria of the Fallopian tube. The

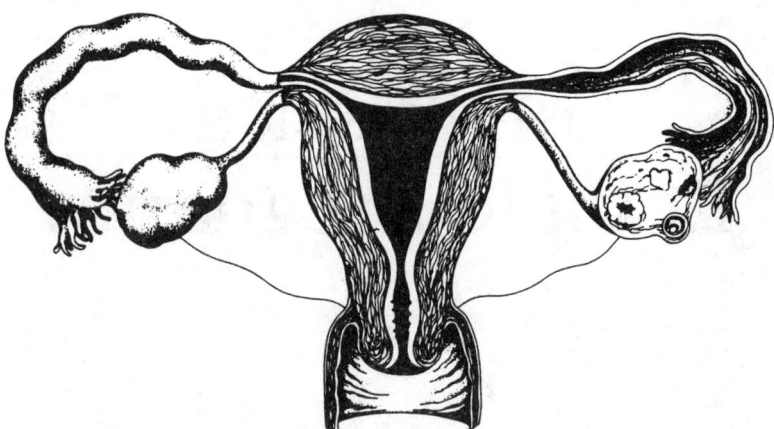

Figure 8.1a *Normal Uterus, Fallopian tubes, and ovaries.*

egg is carried along the channel of the tube and fertilized within the tube. At approximately the midpoint of the tube, the fertilized egg begins to divide and, under normal circumstances, is

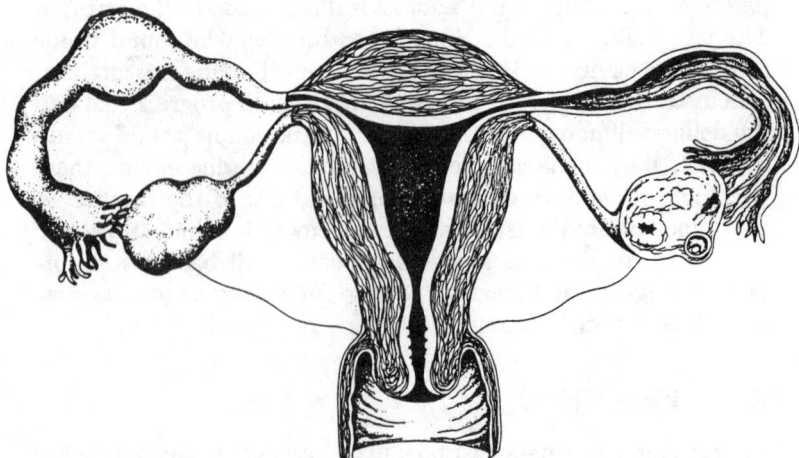

Figure 8.1b *Ectopic Pregnancy located in the middle of the tube—a tubal pregnancy.*

carried along the tube back toward the uterus and into the uterine cavity. The early embryo adheres to the lining of the uterus and begins to grow into a fetus, and eventually a baby. When the fertilized egg is not carried into the uterine cavity but instead allowed to grow in another area, this is referred to as an *extrauterine* or ectopic pregnancy. Other similar terms meaning the same thing are *extrauterine* or *ectopic gestation*. The fertilized egg may get stuck in the Fallopian tube and implant within its wall. Here, the embryo will gradually grow bigger, expanding within the wall of the tube. The tube will begin to stretch and bulge until eventually the embryo will outgrow the structure of the Fallopian tube, causing the tube to tear or rupture. When this happens, the patient may feel a sudden stabbing pain as the tube bursts. Very frequently, sudden heavy bleeding into the abdominal cavity will occur; this is called an *acute intraabdominal hemorrhage*. As the bleeding goes on, there may be a change in blood pressure and the woman may feel dizzy. In extreme cases, she may faint. If this is not treated promptly, the woman may die of sudden extreme blood loss. Such an ectopic pregnancy occurring within the Fallopian tube is called a tubal pregnancy or a *tubal gestation*. Fortunately, death from a ruptured tubal pregnancy is very rare in this country.

The fertilized egg may also implant on a surface other than within the Fallopian tube. This can include the surface of the ovary, resulting in an *ovarian pregnancy*. Much more rarely, the embryo may adhere to almost any surface within the abdominal cavity. Such pregnancies are called *abdominal pregnancies*. A tubal pregnancy may begin to develop in the outer portion of the tube and then may be spontaneously expelled from the end of the tube, resulting in a small amount of bleeding and the death of the embryo. This is called a *tubal abortion*.

WHO IS AT RISK

Approximately 0.5–1.5 percent of women who become pregnant have ectopic pregnancies. There are certain factors associated with an increased risk of tubal pregnancy. Women who have had previous abdominal surgery—including ovarian cyst resections, tubal reconstructions, and surgery for previous ectopic pregnancies—have an increased risk of having an extrauterine pregnancy. Women who have had pelvic infections, including gonorrhea, ureaplasma, and chlamydial infections, have a higher risk of having an ectopic pregnancy. A pelvic infection may be totally without symptoms and still produce enough tubal damage to encourage the development of a tubal pregnancy. Endometriosis, a condition where the tissue that lines the uterine cavity can also be found outside the uterine cavity, is another condition that is associated with tubal pregnancies. Endometriosis can produce tubal scarring that compromises the functioning of the tube and may prevent the movement of the fertilized egg to the uterus.

In vitro fertilization is a process in which an egg is removed from a woman's body, fertilized in the laboratory, and the embryo transferred into the cavity of the woman's uterus. It is often thought that since the embryo is put in the uterus, a tubal pregnancy is not possible. This is not true. In approximately 3–6 percent of pregnancies resulting from *in vitro* fertilization, the embryo can implant itself within the Fallopian tube. This seems to result from the movement of the embryo from the uterine cavity back into the Fallopian tube after it has been properly placed inside the uterus.

No woman who is capable of pregnancy is immune from having an ectopic pregnancy, so even a woman who has had no difficulty in achieving pregnancy must be tested to rule out the possibility of an ectopic pregnancy.

Although 0.5–1.5 percent of the general population will have an ectopic pregnancy, after having had a single ectopic pregnancy, the chances of having a second one increase to 12–15 percent. This still means that the vast majority of women who have had a single ectopic pregnancy will have a normal second pregnancy within the uterus. Nevertheless, if you have had one previous ectopic pregnancy, your doctor must view your second pregnancy with even greater suspicion to be sure it is not a recurrent ectopic pregnancy. After two ectopic pregnancies, the chances of a third increase to 20 percent and after a third, the chance of a fourth ectopic pregnancy increases to 25 percent. As a general rule, after three ectopic pregnancies, the chances that the next pregnancy will occur outside the uterus are greater than that it will be within the uterus: the risk is greater that you will have a dangerous ectopic pregnancy than a safe pregnancy. It is for this reason that we suggest that a woman who has had three ectopic consecutive pregnancies not attempt pregnancy by ordinary means. If pregnancy is still desired, *in vitro* fertilization would be a far safer way of achieving it.

The use of IUDs, having had multiple partners, and being over the age of 35 have been statistically associated with an increased risk of ectopic pregnancy. As the list of possible risk factors associated with ectopic pregnancy grows longer and longer, it might seem as though every pregnant woman can be included in one risk group or another. It then appears that the safest position is to screen every pregnant woman for ectopic pregnancy.

DIAGNOSING AN ECTOPIC PREGNANCY

Probably the most important single factor in diagnosing an ectopic pregnancy is suspicion. Your physician should consider that all pregnant infertility patients—and indeed all pregnant patients—might possibly have a tubal pregnancy. When a woman is pregnant, the placenta produces a hormone called human chorionic gonadotropin, or HCG. This hormone molecule is shaped very much like the letter H, with two parallel lines of the molecule, one called the alpha chain, the other called the beta chain. The beta chain is unique to the HCG molecule. A highly accurate laboratory test has been developed for the beta chain of the HCG molecule. Thus, beta HCG in a blood or urine sample is probably the most sensitive pregnancy test that exists. In most cases, the blood test is more accurate than the urine. Blood levels of HCG should increase by 50–100 percent every $2^{1}/_{2}$ to $3^{1}/_{2}$ days when a woman is thought to be pregnant.

If the laboratory says that HCG is present, then there is a good possibility that the woman is pregnant. The next step is to measure the increasing values of HCG in the blood. Since we know the rate at which HCG levels rise in a healthy pregnancy, this is what we look for. By drawing and testing blood at 3- to 7-day intervals and plotting the HCG levels, you can observe the

HCG levels rising along a predetermined curve. If one blood value falls beneath the curve, that does not mean anything. But if two are beneath the curve, that begins to indicate that the pregnancy is compromised, wherever it is. When the HCG levels reach a certain predetermined level, the embryo should be able to be seen within the uterine cavity by using ultrasound scan. If this value is reached and the ultrasound does not show an embryo within the uterus, the probability of an extrauterine pregnancy becomes very high. The more sophisticated ultrasound becomes, the earlier the diagnosis of ectopic pregnancy can be made.

Ultrasound uses sound waves to visualize the soft tissues of the body, converting those waves into an image on a video screen. This is done by using a small transducer—that sometimes looks like a small flashlight—connected by a cable to a large machine that appears very much like a video screen with a computer attached. The transducer is placed in direct contact with a patient's body and produces sound waves that penetrate her body and bounce back. The transducer picks up the reflected sound waves and converts them to electrical impulses. They are changed by the ultrasound machine into an image. New high-resolution machines allow the production of more precise images to help make the diagnosis of ectopic pregnancy earlier. It is now generally possible to see a sac within the uterus about a week and a half after a missed period.

As HCG levels reach a value of about 6,000 to 6,500, it is usually possible to see the sac surrounding the embryo within the uterine cavity. As ultrasound technology becomes more refined, it might even be possible to make the diagnosis of an intrauterine pregnancy earlier.

Thus the combination of HCG studies and ultrasound scans can be useful in determining the viability of an embryo and its location. Neither of these two techniques definitely diagnoses an ectopic pregnancy. Rising HCG levels tell your physician whether the embryo is doing well or not. There is no characteristic value or rate of rising HCG that indicates an extrauterine pregnancy. What the HCG value does tell the physician is when he or she should be able to see the embryo in the uterus on ultrasound. If an ultrasound scan is done at this time and a sac is not seen within the uterine cavity, there is a high probability that the embryo is somewhere outside the uterus. Having made the diagnosis of a possible ectopic pregnancy, the doctor should then do a laparoscopy to confirm the diagnosis.

A laparoscopy is an operation done while you are under anaesthesia. The surgeon makes an incision in your umbilicus (your belly button) and inserts a telescopelike device into your body to examine the contents of your abdominal cavity, your uterus, and your Fallopian tubes. In this case, laparoscopy can be used to confirm that an embryo exists outside the uterine cavity and to locate it. Sometimes the surgeon can use additional instruments with the laparoscope—passing them through the abdominal wall—to remove the segment of tube that contains the tubal pregnancy or to remove the ectopic pregnancy from the ovary. At other times, the laparoscopy will indicate to the surgeon that a *laparotomy*, regular abdominal surgery, is necessary to treat the extrauterine pregnancy.

TREATMENT

Surgery

The standard treatment for tubal pregnancy has been a *salpingectomy*, the removal of the tube containing the embryo. Removing one Fallopian tube while leaving an apparently normal opposite tube has been associated with a reduction in fertility. For this reason an effort has been made to develop procedures that preserve the tube containing the ectopic pregnancy. Such operations have been successful. One procedure is called a *salpingotomy*. The surgeon makes an incision in the Fallopian tube directly over the embryo and removes the embryo, leaving the tube intact. Another procedure is a *segmental resection*. In this operation, the segment of the tube containing the ectopic pregnancy is removed and the tube can either be reconstructed at the same time or at a later time, if necessary.

Frequently the surgeon removes the segment and ties off the remaining pieces of the Fallopian tube and, if the remaining tube appears to be normal, the couple may attempt pregnancy again. If pregnancy has not occurred within six to twelve cycles, the segments of the tube can be reattached in a standard microsurgical tubal anastomosis (see Chapter 6). Procedures that do not remove the Fallopian tube containing an ectopic pregnancy are called *conservative surgical procedures*.

Drug Treatment

Newer, even more conservative therapy is being developed. Certain drugs can be used to cause the death and absorption of an embryo or pregnancy tissue. One such drug is methotrexate. This drug is used to treat a special form of cancer that develops from pregnancy tissue within the uterus. A number of years ago some Japanese investigators started using methotrexate to treat confirmed tubal pregnancies. Early reports are encouraging, showing that small tubal pregnancies can be absorbed by giving the woman methotrexate. If the tubal gestation is large, methotrexate can be associated with significant bleeding as the embryo dies and passes from the tube.

New technologies must be developed hand in hand. As high-resolution ultrasound continues to improve, it will be possible to make the diagnosis of ectopic pregnancy earlier and more precisely. In the near future, we can look forward to the reliable and very early diagnosis of the location of the embryo, making surgical verification of ectopic pregnancy with a laparoscope unnecessary. The diagnosis of an ectopic pregnancy will be made early, when the total mass of the embryo is small, and before the tube can rupture. Treatment using methotrexate or some other drug will be started and the pregnancy tissue will be absorbed.

Methotrexate is not a harmless drug. It can be associated with changes in liver function and with the reduction of white blood cell count. And so it may be that the ultimate drug used to treat ectopic pregnancy will not be methotrexate but some similar but safer derivative. We do not yet know if the Fallopian tubes of women who have had their tubal pregnancies treated with methotrexate will function normally. We do know that X-rays of these tubes weeks or months later show normal tubal structure. While this is encouraging, it is still not a guarantee that these tubes will function normally and properly. Nevertheless, it is becoming clear that with the combined technology of laboratory studies and ultrasound visualization, ectopic pregnancy is changing from a surgical emergency where treatment must be started because a woman is in shock to a more controlled surgical situation where tubal function can be preserved. In the foreseeable future, it will change to an even more conservative state or will be treated not surgically but with drugs.

In Vitro Fertilization

It may be that the ultimate treatment for repetitive ectopic pregnancies—in terms of maintaining fertility—will be in vitro fertilization. If you have had to have both Fallopian tubes removed or, in spite of conservation therapy, have had three ectopic pregnancies, then in vitro fertilization offers an opportunity for you to achieve pregnancy with a reasonable degree of success at a minimal risk of future extrauterine pregnancy. See Chapter 11 for further discussion of in vitro fertilization.

CHAPTER 9
Endometriosis

THE TISSUE that lines the cavity within the uterus is a mossy material call endometrium that constantly grows and changes throughout a woman's cycle. Occasionally, small pieces of endometrium may be found in other locations in a woman's body. These include the outside surface of the uterus, the Fallopian tubes, the ovaries, the bladder, and, rarely, places distant from the abdominal cavity such as the lung and even the brain. The condition in which apparently normal endometrial tissue is found in locations other than the uterus is called endometriosis. (Figure 9.1.) It is reported to exist in between 7 and 50 percent of all menstruating women, depending on which studies you choose to believe. Some investigators feel that endometriosis is increasing because of the current tendency of women to delay their pregnancies into their middle and late thirties. There is a strong association of endometriosis with infertility. Approximately 30–40 percent of women with endometriosis are unable to achieve a pregnancy. This is approximately twice the incidence of infertility in the general population. On the other hand, this statistic emphasizes that not every woman with endometriosis is infertile. Furthermore, about 6–15 percent of infertile women have endometriosis, making it a very significant cause of infertility. This reduction of fertility is directly related to the extent and severity of the condition.

Just as the endometrium lining the cavity of the uterus re-

Patient's Name _____ Date_____

Stage I (Minimal) · 1-5
Stage II (Mild) · 6-15
Stage III (Moderate) · 16-40
Stage IV (Severe) · >40

Laparoscopy_____ Laparotomy_____ Photography_____
Recommended Treatment_____

Total_____

Prognosis_____

PERITONEUM	**ENDOMETRIOSIS**	<1cm	1-3cm	>3cm
	Superficial	1	2	4
	Deep	2	4	6
OVARY	R Superficial	1	2	4
	Deep	4	16	20
	L Superficial	1	2	4
	Deep	4	16	20

	POSTERIOR CULDESAC OBLITERATION	Partial	Complete
		4	40

	ADHESIONS	<1/3 Enclosure	1/3-2/3 Enclosure	>2/3 Enclosure
OVARY	R Filmy	1	2	4
	Dense	4	8	16
	L Filmy	1	2	4
	Dense	4	8	16
TUBE	R Filmy	1	2	4
	Dense	4*	8*	16
	L Filmy	1	2	4
	Dense	4*	8*	16

*If the fimbriated end of the fallopian tube is completely enclosed, change the point assignment to 16.

Additional Endometriosis: _____

Associated Pathology: _____

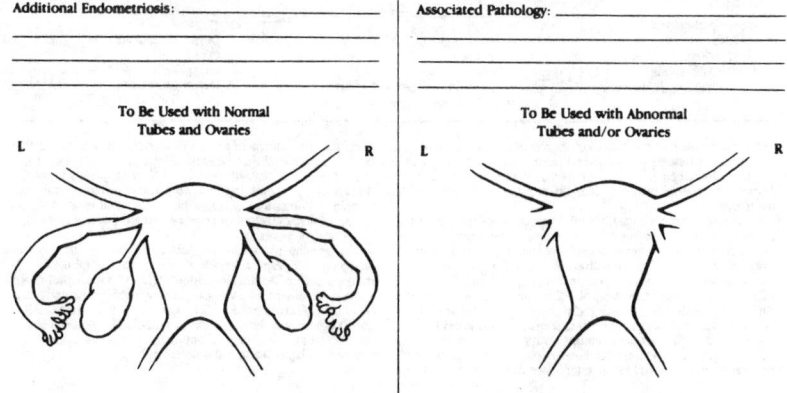

To Be Used with Normal
Tubes and Ovaries

L   R

To Be Used with Abnormal
Tubes and/or Ovaries

L   R

For additional supply write to: The American Fertility Society, 2131 Magnolia Avenue,
Suite 201, Birmingham, Alabama 35256

Figure 9.1a and b *The American Fertility Society's classification of endometriosis.*

EXAMPLES & GUIDELINES

STAGE I (MINIMAL) | STAGE II (MILD) | STAGE III (MODERATE)

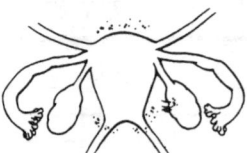 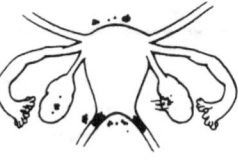 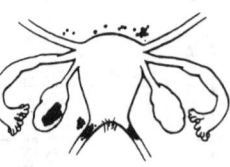

PERITONEUM
  Superficial Endo – 1-3cm · 2
R. OVARY
  Superficial Endo – < 1cm · 1
  Filmy Adhesions – < 1/3 · 1
  TOTAL POINTS 4

PERITONEUM
  Deep Endo – >3cm · 6
R. OVARY
  Superficial Endo – < 1cm · 1
  Filmy Adhesions – < 1/3 · 1
L. OVARY
  Superficial Endo – < 1cm · 1
  TOTAL POINTS 9

PERITONEUM
  Deep Endo – >3cm · 6
CULDESAC
  Partial Obliteration · 4
L. OVARY
  Deep Endo – 1-3cm · 16
  TOTAL POINTS 26

STAGE III (MODERATE) | STAGE IV (SEVERE) | STAGE IV (SEVERE)

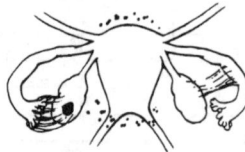 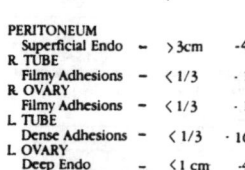 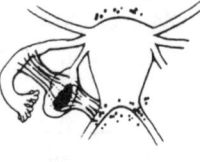 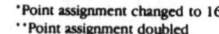 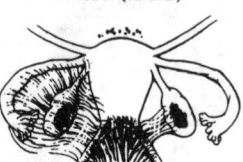

PERITONEUM
  Superficial Endo – >3cm -4
R. TUBE
  Filmy Adhesions – < 1/3 · 1
R. OVARY
  Filmy Adhesions – < 1/3 · 1
L. TUBE
  Dense Adhesions – < 1/3 · 16*
L. OVARY
  Deep Endo – <1 cm -4
  Dense Adhesions – < 1/3 -4
  TOTAL POINTS 30

PERITONEUM
  Superficial Endo – >3cm -4
L. OVARY
  Deep Endo – 1-3cm · 32**
  Dense Adhesions – < 1/3 · 8**
L. TUBE
  Dense Adhesions – < 1/3 · 8**
  TOTAL POINTS 52

*Point assignment changed to 16
**Point assignment doubled

PERITONEUM
  Deep Endo – >3cm · 6
CULDESAC
  Complete Obliteration · 40
R. OVARY
  Deep Endo – 1-3cm · 16
  Dense Adhesions – < 1/3 · 4
L. TUBE
  Dense Adhesions – >2/3 · 16
L. OVARY
  Deep Endo – 1-3cm · 16
  Dense Adhesions – >2/3 · 16
  TOTAL POINTS 114

Determination of the stage or degree of endometrial involvement is based on a weighted point system. Distribution of points has been arbitrarily determined and may require further revision or refinement as knowledge of the disease increases.

To ensure complete evaluation, inspection of the pelvis in a clockwise or counterclockwise fashion is encouraged. Number, size and location of endometrial implants, plaques, endometriomas and/or adhesions are noted. For example, five separate 0.5cm superficial implants on the peritoneum (2.5 cm total) would be assigned 2 points. (The surface of the uterus should be considered peritoneum.) The severity of the endometriosis or adhesions should be assigned the highest score only for peritoneum, ovary, tube or culdesac. For example, a 4cm superficial and a 2cm deep implant of the peritoneum should be given a score of 6 (not 8). A 4cm

deep endometrioma of the ovary associated with more than 3cm of superficial disease should be scored 20 (not 24).

In those patients with only one adnexa, points applied to disease of the remaining tube and ovary should be multiplied by two. **Points assigned may be circled and totaled. Aggregation of points indicates stage of disease (minimal, mild, moderate, or severe).

The presence of endometriosis of the bowel, urinary tract, fallopian tube, vagina, cervix, skin etc., should be documented under "additional endometriosis." Other pathology such as tubal occlusion, leiomyomata, uterine anomaly, etc., should be documented under "associated pathology." All pathology should be depicted as specifically as possible on the sketch of pelvic organs, and means of observation (laparoscopy or laparotomy) should be noted.

sponds to the change in normal output of the ovary during the course of your cycle, so does the misplaced endometrial tissue forming the implants of endometriosis. When it is time for the tissue within your uterus to crumble and be shed—forming your menstrual period—the implants of endometriosis also break down. But since there is no exit for this crumbling material to use, the materials produced by the breakdown of the endometrial tissue migrate into the tissue surrounding the implant. Some of the substances released by the endometrium are called *prostaglandins*. When the endometrium within the uterus releases prostaglandins, they migrate into the uterine muscle, causing the tissue to cramp, producing menstrual cramps. When prostaglandins migrate into the tissue surrounding an implant of endometriosis, they irritate this tissue. Because the tissue is constantly and repeatedly irritated, it becomes damaged and is replaced by scar tissue. It is very common for endometriosis to be associated with intense pain at the time of a woman's period and significant scar tissue production. The scar tissue may directly surround the implanted endometriosis and/or may form bands of adhesions extending from the surface of the implant to neighboring organ surfaces. Thus it is possible for endometriosis to be associated with infertility on a mechanical basis resulting from scar tissue production. For instance, these bands of scar tissue or adhesions can form a web around the Fallopian tube or tubes, preventing proper egg pickup.

Reduction of fertility from endometriosis is statistically directly related to the extent of the disease. With severe endometriosis there is usually extensive adhesion formation and scarring around the implants, involving the ovaries and Fallopian tubes. Here the mechanism of infertility appears obvious: the scar tissue interferes with egg pickup and tubal functioning. However, in cases of minimal endometriosis, small implants of this tissue can be present on the bladder, on the front of the uterus, or in some location far from the ovary or Fallopian tubes and still be associated with infertility. It then becomes clear that the mechanism by which endometriosis causes infertility is more than simply the production of scar tissue.

One of the more fascinating things about endometriosis is that it is a condition of contradictions. There is nothing that can be said about the disease that uniformly applies to everyone who has it. For example, not every woman with endometriosis is infertile, nor does everyone who has this condition have pain with her periods. Sometimes endometriosis is unexpectedly found at the time of cesarean section in women who had no difficulty in becoming pregnant and who never experienced any menstrual discomfort.

WHAT CAUSES IT

Medical science generally believes that endometriosis is the result of what is called "retrograde menstruation." At the time of a woman's menses, the endometrium within the uterus crumbles and is shed through the vagina. Some of this endometrial tissue may not drain out of the uterus during menstruation. Instead, it may back up into the Fallopian tubes and escape into the abdominal cavity where it may begin to grow on the surfaces on which it settles. It is believed that 50 percent of all women have significant retrograde menstruation. However, most of these women do not develop endometriosis. Why do some women develop such foci of growing tissue, while others, despite continued retrograde menstruation, do not?

Some investigators have studied the occurrence of endometriosis in the relatives of women with endometriosis as well as in unrelated women. These studies have shown that the immediate female relatives of a woman with endometriosis have a higher than expected incidence of endometriosis. Furthermore, the severity of endometriosis also seems to be increased within a family tree; both the incidence and the severity of endometriosis are genetically influenced. The association is not an absolute one; if endometriosis is found in one member of a family, it does not guarantee that all others will have it. However, the association is greater than we would expect randomly. Some investigators feel that the transmission of endometriosis is possibly due to the combination of several genes or to a composite of both genetic and environmental factors.

One environmental factor is the total amount of endometrial

tissue delivered into the abdominal cavity by retrograde menstruation, as is made clear by the incidence of endometriosis in women with uterine abnormalities in which the outflow of menstrual blood is completely obstructed. Here, virtually all of the endometrium pours into the abdominal cavity rather than out through the vagina. The incidence of endometriosis in these women is extremely high.

Thus the development of endometriotic implants in some patients depends upon the retrograde flow of the endometrial cells from the uterine cavity. When the amount of such tissue is delivered in a high volume and frequency, then most women develop endometriosis. When the volume or frequency is low, fewer patients develop endometriosis and its development may very well be a reflection of a genetic predisposition.

Endometriosis is also associated with ovulation abnormalities. Some studies have shown that 17–27 percent of infertile women with endometriosis do not ovulate, and 25–45 percent with endometriosis have progesterone deficiencies. Some investigators' data shows that as many as 79 percent of women with endometriosis have Luteinized Unruptured Follicle syndrome.

Luteinized Unruptured Follicle syndrome is a condition in which the follicle containing the egg goes through all the proper changes prior to ovulation but the actual release of the egg never takes place. The follicle then converts to a corpus luteum producing progesterone, usually in normal amounts, but with the egg still trapped within it. The result is that many, if not all, of the hormonal studies consistent with ovulation are normal, but pregnancy does not occur because the egg is never released.

It should be noted that all of these ovulatory abnormalities—the absence of ovulation, progesterone deficiency, as well as the luteinized unruptured follicle—can be treated with conventional ovulation induction agents such as clomiphene and/or Pergonal.

Endometriosis has also been associated with poor sperm survival in the woman's reproductive tract. Poor postcoital tests occur more frequently in women with endometriosis than in the general infertile population. A woman can take certain drugs to increase the chances of sperm survival in these cases.

From all of this data it becomes clear that endometriosis is more than misplaced bits of endometrial tissue. Endometriosis appears to produce infertility by a variety of mechanisms. It can generate local scar tissue, forming adhesions that entrap the Fallopian tube and making egg pickup difficult to impossible. Scar tissue on the wall of the Fallopian tube may destroy its muscle and its lining, preventing the tube from functioning normally. Endometriosis can also be associated with ovulation abnormalities. These can be nonovulation (anovulation), irregular ovulation, progesterone deficiencies and/or Luteinized Unruptured Follicle syndrome. Another possible cause of infertility can be poor sperm survival within the female reproductive tract. The mechanism of this is not clear but the treatment appears to be straightforward.

Some investigators have described an increase in miscarriage rate in women who have gotten pregnant with untreated endometriosis. When the endometriosis is treated either with drugs or by surgery, the miscarriage rate diminishes to that of the general population. It may very well be that some of the infertility ascribed to endometriosis is really very early miscarriage that occurs even before a positive pregnancy test is obtained.

DIAGNOSIS

Since there are many problems associated with endometriosis, the treatment should be a broad spectrum form of therapy. If you have endometriosis, your doctor should concentrate on more than simply treating the implants of tissue. Your doctor diagnoses endometriosis by laparoscopy. You are admitted to a hospital and taken to an operating room, where anesthesia is administered. The surgeon makes a small incision in your umbilicus—your navel—then inserts a laparoscope into the abdomen and looks at its contents. Through this telescope, the surgeon can see small brown implants—which look very much like bits of cigarette tobacco—sticking to various surfaces within the abdominal cavity. Each one of these small implants is endometriosis. The areas are frequently surrounded by a whitish halo of tissue, the surrounding fibrous tissue produced by the migration of prostaglandin into the normal tissue. Sometimes bands of dense fibers can be seen projecting from these implants—like spokes from a wheel—attaching themselves to the surrounding tissue. These bands are areas of adhesions. Occasionally the areas of endometriosis can be large areas of fibrous tissue that cause the tubes and ovaries to adhere to one another. When all these structures form one large mass as if glue had been poured into the pelvis, the condition is called a *frozen pelvis*. This represents one extreme that can result from misplaced endometrial tissue. Endometriosis may also form bubblelike structures filled with chocolate-like, pasty material on the surface of the ovary. These ovarian cysts containing endometriosis are referred to as *endometriomata* (one cyst is called an *endometrioma*).

TREATMENT

Surgery

Using a laparoscope, a surgeon can evaluate the extent of the disease. Sometimes by making an additional incision in your abdomen and introducing one or two more instruments, the surgeon can vaporize the endometriosis implants. The endometrial tissue can be destroyed by using one of several kinds of lasers or electric current. Whether or not this can be done successfully depends on how much endometriosis is present and what the underlying structures are. If the structures immediately beneath the areas of endometriosis are blood vessels, intestines, or other vital structures that may be damaged by the vaporization process, then it is probably not safe or prudent to carry out such a procedure through laparoscopic surgery. In this case, full abdominal surgery can be used. Using electric current, lasers, or conventional surgery, areas of endometriosis can be cut out. Care must be taken in doing this to try to minimize trauma to neighboring tissues.

The probability of success following surgery depends on the extent of the disease. The American Fertility Society has offered a classification of endometriosis. (Figure 9.1a and 9.2b.) Points

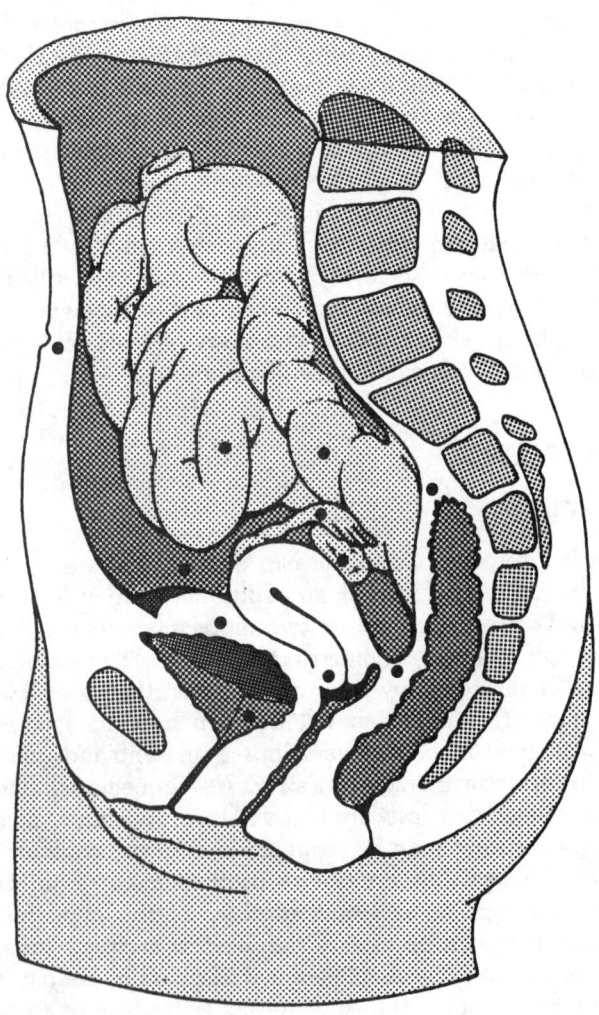

Figure 9.2 *Endometriosis. Some of the possible sites of endometriosis are shown.*

are given for the amount of endometriosis present and what tissue it involves. The greater the total number of points, the poorer the surgical outcome.

Drug Treatment

Endometrial tissue requires estrogen in order to survive. If we could cut off the estrogen supply to this tissue, the endometrium would shrivel up or, in medical terms, become atrophic. Since estrogen is predominantly produced by the ovary and the ovary in turn is stimulated by the FSH and LH from the pituitary, we have a possible mechanism of treating endometriosis. If there were a drug which would turn off FSH and LH production, estrogen levels would drop and the endometrium, wherever it might be, would atrophy. The result would be that the lining of the uterus would become quite thin and the implants of endometriosis might shrivel up even more. In fact, this is exactly what does happen with drug treatment.

If an oral contraceptive is given to a woman, FSH and LH production are dramatically reduced and endometriosis frequently becomes suppressed. However, since most oral contraceptives contain estrogen, a certain amount of estrogen stimulus is given to the tissue. Because of this, another form of treatment—called pseudomenopause—has evolved. With this form of treatment, a drug not containing estrogen is given to suppress FSH and LH production. Estrogen levels fall and the endometrial implants become atrophic. Since there is no estrogen available from either the drug or the ovary, the degree of suppression of endometriosis is greater than that achieved with oral contraceptive treatment.

There are three forms of treatment available for pseudomenopause. The first and most commonly used is Danocrine (the generic name is danazol). This drug is a derivative of a male hormone that has had most of its male properties stripped from it. It suppresses FSH and LH production quite well and is usually given in doses of 200 to 800 milligrams a day for three to six months or for nine months. At higher doses it suppresses ovarian function and ovulation and reduces the size of endometrial implants. It is usually not successful in treating significant endo-metrioma. The advantage of danazol therapy is that it allows endometriosis to be treated without the risks of surgery, including the possibility of causing damage to underlying structures and the risks of anesthesia. The disadvantage of danazol therapy is the possibility of drug reactions. Since the goal of this therapy is to produce a pseudomenopausal state, women taking danazol will usually not have regular periods. The drug reduces estrogen levels, suppressing the growth of endometrium and affecting the lining of the uterus as significantly as the implants of endometriosis. The lining of the uterus becomes progressively thinner and may crack and bleed irregularly. Irregular vaginal staining or bleeding is not uncommon with danazol therapy—in a sense it is a good sign because it reflects to some degree the suppression of the lining of the uterus. The suppression parallels the atrophy of the implants of endometriosis. Women may also notice a decrease in breast size as well as hot flushes, popularly called "hot flashes," which are both related to the reduction of estrogen levels. The cycles of a woman taking danazol usually return to normal about six weeks after she stops taking the drug. Breast size also returns to normal.

Other side effects may be related to male hormone effects of the drug, with acne and hair growth occasionally occurring. In very rare cases, your voice may deepen. This effect is not reversible, but it is virtually always preceded by a huskiness of the voice that is reversible. If you are on danazol you should let your physician know if you notice a marked huskiness of your voice. At this point, your doctor will usually discontinue the drug and substitute a new one.

This description makes danazol sound like a terrible drug with horrible and unacceptable side effects. In fact, it is usually well tolerated and its effect on endometriosis can be very dramatic. Pregnancy rates in properly selected women can be as high as 75 percent.

Another drug that can be used to treat endometriosis is medroxyprogesterone (marketed in the United States under the name Provera). Medroxyprogesterone, given in a tablet form of 30 to 50 milligrams per day, can have an effect that is very much like that of danazol. It too suppresses FSH and LH production and results in the atrophy of endometrial implants. Many of its side effects are similar to danazol's, except that medroxyprogesterone is a derivative not of a male hormone but of progesterone, and therefore has none of danazol's male hormone side effects. As such, medroxyprogesterone is not associated with the appearance of acne, male pattern hair growth, or deepening of the voice. Medroxyprogesterone can suppress endometriosis as well as danazol, but pregnancy rates are slightly less than danazol's, which is why most doctors first try danazol.

Another drug that is just now being tested in the United States but is already used in other countries is the whole class of GnRH analogues. (See Chapter 12.) These drugs, which are administered either by injection or by nasal spray, act on the pituitary to turn off FSH and LH production. Their effect on endometriosis can be very dramatic; early reports seem to show that they are more effective than either of the two drugs described above and may even be successful at shrinking endometriomata. Since they are not derivatives of any of the usual hormone classes, male changes—appearance of acne, male pattern hair growth, and deepening of the voice—do not occur. There is not enough evidence at this time to say whether these drugs will be the "magic bullet" to treat endometriosis, but the early experience appears to be very positive.

All of these drugs only suppress endometriosis; they do nothing for the scar tissue. They also do nothing to treat the other associated problems that can exist with endometriosis—ovulatory problems, sperm survival problems, and so on. If scar tissue plays a major role in preventing pregnancy, then drug-induced suppression of endometriosis will not be enough; surgery may be necessary. There are times when a combination of drug treatment and surgery will be called for.

We never speak of curing endometriosis: it tends to recur even after the most aggressive drug treatment and/or surgery. Nevertheless, endometriosis may not recur until after you become pregnant.

After the areas of endometriosis have been removed by surgery or drug treatment, and the scar tissue removed by surgery, if necessary, then you may begin treatment for ovulatory abnormalities and sperm survival problems. Ovulation defects can be treated with Clomid, Pergonal, or progesterone, according to the particular problem that exists. Sperm survival can often be enhanced by small doses of prednisone. It is probably counterproductive to treat poor cervical mucus in any women with endometriosis by giving her estrogen.

If all appropriate therapy has been tried without achieving a pregnancy, in vitro fertilization is an excellent choice. It should be noted that in vitro fertilization is associated with slightly reduced success when performed on women with endometriosis. Nevertheless, it may very well be the best way for a woman with endometriosis who has already been treated appropriately and has not achieved a pregnancy, to become pregnant. For further discussion of in vitro fertilization, see Chapter 11.

CHAPTER 10
DES Sons and Daughters

In the late 1940s and early 1950s, medical science believed that a pregnancy in danger of being lost could be saved by administering a drug called diethylstilbestrol, known as DES, to the pregnant mother. Following DES treatment, many pregnancies continued uneventfully while others did not survive. Later studies showed that the administration of DES did not increase the chances of survival of these pregnancies. In 1971 the Food and Drug Administration banned the use of DES in pregnancy. That same year Arthur Herbst reported finding a rare form of vaginal cancer, clear-cell adenocarcinoma, in some women exposed to DES while fetuses in their mothers' uteri.

The result of this therapy was the exposure of two groups of people to diethylstilbestrol. One group consists of pregnant mothers who took the drug themselves. This group is generally referred to as "DES mothers." The second group is composed of the offspring of these pregnancies—the sons and daughters of DES mothers who were exposed to diethylstilbestrol while still in their mother's body. Frequently, these men and women are referred to as "DES sons and daughters." It is estimated that up to 1.5 million women were exposed to DES before birth.

In 1977, Raymond Kaufman published a paper describing abnormalities of the uterine cavity that had not been seen before. The women in whom these observations were made were DES daughters. Dr. Kaufman suggested that the impaired reproduc-

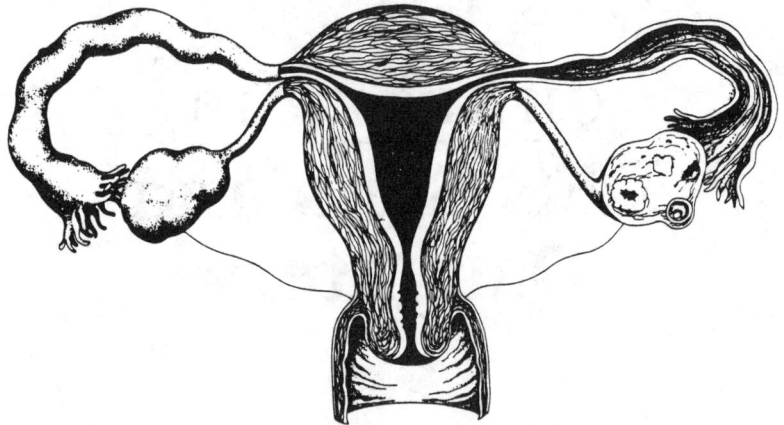

Figure 10.1a *Normal uterus, uterine cavity, and cervix.*

tive ability of the women studied was related to the uterine abnormalities described.

Physicians are always concerned about the possible effect of any drug taken by a pregnant woman on her developing fetus. Up to the time of the discovery of abnormalities in DES offspring, doctors felt that if a fetal abnormality were to be produced by drug exposure during pregnancy, that abnormality would be visible at the time of the baby's birth. DES represented the first known cause of abnormalities associated with fetal drug exposure which were not obvious at the time of delivery but appeared to develop later in life. DES daughters did not have the observable findings until their teenage years.

Further evaluations showed that DES daughters have a number of abnormalities in common, including abnormalities of the cervix and the shape of the uterine cavity. Most women have a uterine cavity that is shaped very much like a triangle; (Figure 10.1a) DES daughters have a uterine cavity that is shaped very much like the letter T. This configuration appears to be associated with an increased risk of miscarriage, premature labor, and ectopic pregnancy. The quality of the Fallopian tubes also seems

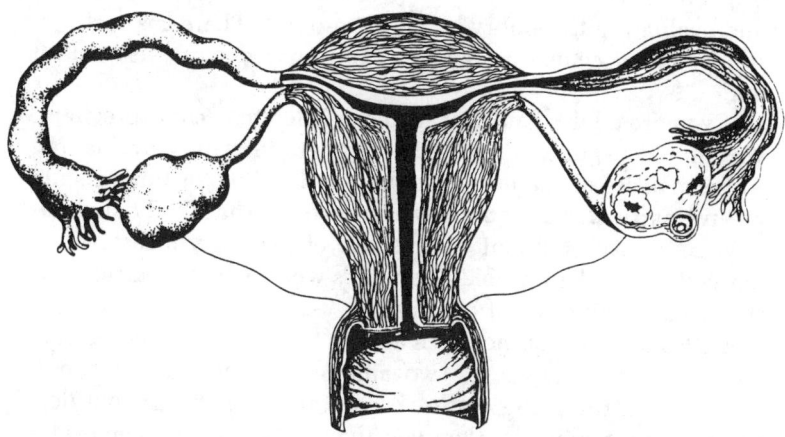

Figure 10.1b *Uterus with a T-shaped uterine cavity and a shortened cervix frequently seen in DES daughters.*

to be affected by DES exposure. DES daughters seem to have slightly narrower, finer tubes.

DES sons sometimes have abnormalities of their ductal system, the network of tubing connecting the testicle to the penis. The result is that there may be diminished sperm production.

DES daughters also have changes in cervical mucus production so that sperm survival during intercourse may be diminished. The net result is that DES sons and daughters may have difficulties in achieving pregnancy, and, in the case of women, difficulties in carrying a pregnancy once they conceive. It must be strongly emphasized that not all DES offspring have reproductive problems. DES daughters who achieve pregnancy may miscarry, but with each succeeding pregnancy, the survival tends to be better, allowing the pregnancy to go longer and longer.

In DES daughters who continue to attempt pregnancy in spite of recurrent miscarriage, the probability of eventually delivering a living newborn is high. As a DES daughter who becomes pregnant, you have to be thoroughly evaluated. Your doctor should examine each pregnancy for its progress, following HCG values and evaluating the embryo with ultrasound. There is a real possibility of an ectopic pregnancy, and your doctor must rule it out.

If you are a DES daughter who has failed to become pregnant, you should begin a careful and complete infertility evaluation. Abnormalities of the uterus, cervix, and Fallopian tubes should receive particular attention. We have found that DES daughters have an unexpectedly high incidence of poor sperm survival on postcoital test. This problem responds well to drugs, particularly the use of small doses of prednisone.

A DES son who has not been able to father a pregnancy should have a semen analysis. If two analyses are normal, then it is unlikely that the DES exposure caused any problem. If your doctor finds abnormalities, then you should start a complete evaluation of male infertility.

Not all DES sons and daughters have reproductive problems. Those who have difficulty achieving a pregnancy do not necessarily have problems caused by DES exposure. Those whose infertility appears to be related to the drug exposure can be treated and can probably get pregnant. No one can guarantee that any individual will achieve a pregnancy, but without trying and treatment, if necessary, no one can say that he or she has given it his or her best shot.

CHAPTER 11
In Vitro Fertilization

In 1978, an infant girl was delivered in England whose very existence would change the course of human reproduction forever. Her name was Louise Brown and, like any other child, she was the product of the union of her parents' egg and sperm. What made this infant different was that for the first time in human history, a child was formed through fertilization that took place outside the human body—in a test tube. Thus, she was hailed as "the world's first test-tube baby." She represented a new way of achieving pregnancy for those women who had hopelessly blocked Fallopian tubes and who were otherwise unable to achieve pregnancy. Her birth was the result of extensive work done in England by Patrick Steptoe and Robert Edwards. Several other research groups throughout the world had been working on similar projects. Soon after the birth of Louise Brown, pregnancies occurred in Melbourne, Australia, from the Monash University group headed by Carl Wood and Alan Trounson, and later in the United States in Norfolk, Virginia, by Howard Jones' group at Eastern Virginia Medical School. The importance of these events is that the initial success in England was not just a fluke. In science we have learned that many wonderful things have been done—but some only once. Their significance is lost because the work cannot be duplicated. The birth of a child conceived in a test tube was not a laboratory quirk, a once-in-a-lifetime miracle, but something that was verifiable, reproducible, and real.

The terms applied to this miracle are *in vitro fertilization* and *embryo transfer.* "In vitro fertilization" means "fertilization in glass," implying that fertilization has taken place outside the human body in a structure other than the female reproductive system. In vitro does not necessarily mean that fertilization took place in a glass object; the term "glass" is simply used to conjure up visions of a laboratory.

Once fertilization has occurred, the egg begins to divide and develop into a very early embryo. In theory, the embryo could be raised in the laboratory or returned to the mother's uterus or womb. Because the technology of growing an embryo in a laboratory is far more complicated than returning the tiny embryo to the uterus, the choice is simple. The embryo is returned to the uterus and this procedure is referred to as embryo transfer. Since "in vitro fertilization and embryo transfer" is a mouthful to say, write, and read, it is frequently abbreviated simply as IVF/ET or simply IVF.

AN OVERVIEW

Basically, the concept of in vitro fertilization is fairly straightforward. A woman's eggs are contained within her ovaries. In each cycle, one or more eggs ripen, each within its own bubble-like structure called a follicle. Ordinarily, the follicle bursts, releasing an egg, which is picked up by the Fallopian tube. If intercourse occurs at this time, the sperm cells are deposited in the vagina, swim through the cervix into the uterus and into the Fallopian tube where the egg is waiting. It is within the Fallopian tube that fertilization usually takes place and the egg begins to divide. The fertilized egg is carried down the Fallopian tube back into the uterus where it adheres to the lining of the uterine cavity as an early embryo.

In vitro fertilization is a means of bypassing the Fallopian tube entirely. In theory, all one has to do is remove a ripe egg from its follicle, place it in the proper environment, and introduce sperm so that fertilization can take place. After fertilization has occurred, the newly fertilized egg, which has begun to divide, is transferred into the uterus to continue its development (Figure

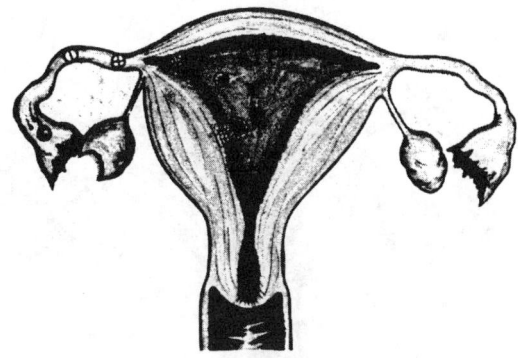

Normal ovulation, fertilization and implantation.
The egg is released from a follicle, picked up by the Fallopian tube, and fertilization occurs in the tube. Three days later, the resulting embryo is moved through the tube into the uterus. The embryo may implant in the uterine lining within the next few days and continue to grow forming a baby.

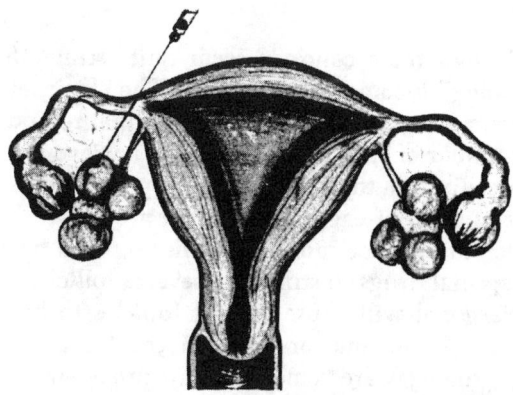

Egg retrieval
If the tubes are blocked and cannot transport the egg from the ovary, IVF can be used to allow egg retrieval from the many follicles stimulated on the ovary for IVF. The eggs are then placed with sperm in test tube. Fertilization occurs there; early embryo development begins.

Figure 11.1 *(Pp. 177–178) General scheme of in vitro fertilization. (Illustrations courtesy of IVF America.)*

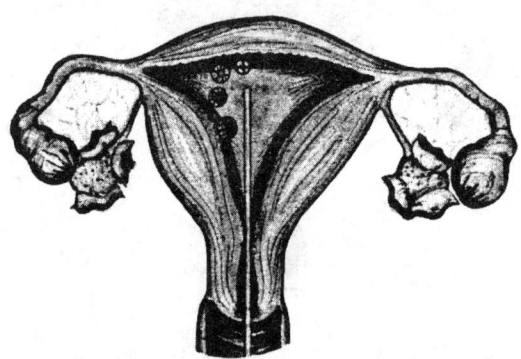

Transfer & Implantation
Two days later, the embryo is transferred into the uterus through a thin catheter placed through the cervix. The embryo may implant in the uterine lining within the next few days.

11.1). Though these concepts seem quite straightforward, the actual "doing" is somewhat complex. The efficiency of the artificial system is not as good as that of normal reproduction. So a greater number of tries are necessary to achieve a pregnancy by in vitro fertilization than by ordinary reproduction and therefore a greater number of eggs per cycle are needed.

In order to produce more than one egg at a time, a woman is given special drugs to stimulate several follicles. Clomiphene and/or Pergonal will cause several follicles to begin to develop at once. When one or more of the follicles contain mature eggs, the eggs are removed. This procedure is called "egg retrieval."

It is critical to perform egg retrieval when one can get as many mature eggs as possible. Immature eggs cannot be fertilized as well and therefore have less chance of producing a pregnancy. If one waits too long, the mature eggs may be released from the surface of the ovary and lost somewhere in the abdominal cavity. Thus, the in vitro team has to walk a very fine line to collect as many mature eggs as possible at the proper time to ensure the greatest chance of success.

There are ways to assess the development and maturity of the developing follicles and the eggs. As the follicles grow, they produce estrogen. The size of the follicle and the amount of estrogen released correspond to the degree of development and maturation of the egg. Physicians take advantage of these two parameters to follow the development and maturation of the egg to determine the precise time that egg retrieval should occur. During the time that a woman is given clomiphene and/or Pergonal, her doctor will take daily blood samples to measure blood estrogen levels. These values should increase daily, representing the development of the follicles. When the values reach a certain predetermined level, ultrasound scans are used to measure the diameter of the developing follicles.

Ultrasound uses sound waves transmitted through the abdominal wall and reflected off the contents of the abdomen. When these sound waves return, they are reconstructed as visual images on a video screen. These images allow us to actually see a cross-section of the ovary and take precise measurements of each follicle. If these measurements are done consecutively, every other day or daily, we can actually chart the growth and development of the follicles visually. When the estrogen levels and the ultrasound both describe one or more mature follicles, the woman is given an injection of HCG. HCG usually triggers ovulation approximately thirty-six hours after its injection. In this way, the exact time of ovulation can be controlled and egg retrieval can be scheduled precisely before ovulation occurs.

Approximately thirty-six hours after the HCG injection, the patient is taken to the operating room where egg retrieval takes place. There are two ways of collecting eggs. One is by laparoscopy, frequently called a *surgical retrieval*. A second, newer technique uses ultrasound and is a *nonsurgical technique*, discussed in detail later in this chapter. With the laparoscopic procedure the patient is taken to an operating room, anesthetized, and a small incision is made in her abdomen at or near the navel, where a laparoscope is inserted. Through the laparoscope, the surgeon can see the uterus and tubes and precisely locate the ripe follicles on each ovary. The surgeon makes the second incision, usually in the midline of the abdomen, about the level of the upper edge of the pubic hairline. Through this tiny incision he or she inserts a long needle and, with laparoscopic guidance, uses the needle to puncture a follicle. The surgeon puts the needle into this bubblelike structure, and carefully draws out the contents and immediately sends them to a nearby laboratory for microscopic examination. The fluid drawn, called *follicular fluid*, usually contains an egg.

A person in the adjacent laboratory, usually an embryologist, scans the fluid to ensure that the egg has been successfully retrieved and that it is mature and then places it in an appropriate culture medium as quickly as possible. This procedure is repeated until all the follicles have been tapped and each egg is in a separate dish. Immature eggs are placed in a different medium in an attempt to allow them to mature in an incubator. Mature eggs or those that have been allowed to ripen in an incubator are allowed to adapt to the incubator environment for approximately six hours.

During this time, the man has been asked to produce a sperm sample. The sperm cells are washed with the culture medium and the most actively moving cells are collected and used for the later steps in the IVF procedure.

This enriched sperm specimen is then introduced into each culture dish containing an egg. In this way, fertilization is allowed to take place. Not every egg that is collected is fertilized. The percentage of eggs that are successfully fertilized varies from laboratory to laboratory and may approach 80 percent.

The embryos are transferred into the woman's uterus by placing them in a long, narrow, plastic tube which the doctor inserts through the cervix. It has been approximately forty-eight hours from the time of fertilization to the time of reinsertion or embryo transfer. This time is variable and will probably change as research continues to refine the best time for the transfer of the embryo. Your doctor places the plastic tube in the uterine cavity and then uses a small syringe on its outside portion to inject the embryo into the uterus.

Pregnancy rates until recently were generally considered to be approximately 15–20 percent per cycle. On the basis of continued development of the procedure, as an example the IVF America program at United Hospital in Port Chester, N.Y. is currently running between a 20 and 25 percent rate per retrieval.

The vast majority of those who enter an in vitro program respond to medication with the development of one or more follicles. Most of those women have successful egg collections with the retrieval of at least one and usually three or more eggs. The majority of the eggs recovered are fertilized and develop into early embryos. However, a relatively small fraction of the embryos that are transferred into the uterus go on to develop into viable, successful pregnancies. Over the next few years, much of the current research will focus on improving the success in this area.

WHAT ACTUALLY HAPPENS

Hormone Stimulation

Here is what a couple will actually experience while going through in vitro fertilization. The woman takes clomiphene, usually two tablets (100 milligrams) for five days starting on the second, third, fourth, or fifth day of her cycle. She will start receiving Pergonal, a drug given in a series of daily injections, usually on the day following the first dose of clomiphene. On the morning of about the fourth day of treatment, a nurse or technician draws the woman's blood to test for estrogen levels. The results are available on the afternoon of the same day. Pergonal is given that day and again the following day, and each morning thereafter blood samples are drawn for estrogen evaluation. The doctors can determine the patient's response to Pergonal stimulation by studying the increase in the daily estrogen levels. Using these blood studies, the doctors can control precisely the amount of stimulation that the patient receives. If the estrogen levels are rising too slowly, Pergonal is increased; if the values are rising too rapidly, the dose of Pergonal can be decreased. When the estrogen levels reach a certain point, ultrasound scans are begun. Usually this is around cycle day six, seven, or eight. The doctors use the combined information of blood estrogen levels, ultrasound measurements of follicular development, and sometimes, physical examination of the woman, to continually watch the development of the follicles and determine the time of the egg's ripeness. An effort is always made to ripen three or more follicles, since an optimum pregnancy rate appears to be associated with the transfer of three or four embryos back into the uterus. When all of the measuring parameters indicate that ideally three or more follicles are ripe, the woman is given an injection of HCG and scheduled for retrieval approximately thirty-six hours later.

All of the procedures done up to this time can be done on an outpatient basis. Hospitalization is not necessary for the administration or monitoring of Pergonal.

Egg Retrieval

At the appropriate time, the woman goes into a hospital and is anesthetized for a laparoscopy. Laparoscopy is a surgical procedure done in an operating room with general anesthesia. Using the laparoscope for guidance, the surgeon inserts a needle through the abdomen and retrieves as many eggs as possible. The eggs are sent to the egg culturing laboratory as soon as they are removed, even before the patient is awakened. When the laparoscopy is completed, the patient is taken to the recovery room and within a short time is discharged from the hospital. Only a brief hospitalization—several hours—is required.

Producing the Sperm Sample

Shortly after the eggs are collected, the man is asked to produce a sperm specimen. Technicians mix the sperm sample with a tissue culture solution and remove the sperm cells from the remainder of the seminal fluid (the fluid in which sperm are produced). They then place the new suspension of sperm cells at the bottom of a special test tube. The sperm cells are allowed to swim toward the top. The healthiest and most actively swimming cells will travel to the top of the solution while the nonmotile (nonmoving) or sluggishly moving cells remain at the bottom. By removing the top layer of the fluid, the technicians in the laboratory are able to obtain a specimen of sperm cells of unusually high quality. Using this tech-

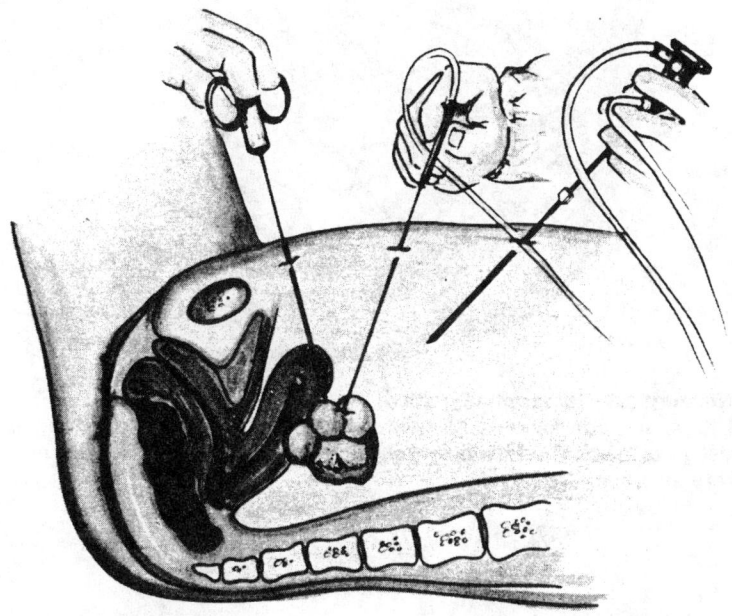

Surgically (laparoscopy)

Laparoscopy is a minor surgical procedure that allows a telescope to be placed through a small incision in the umbilicus. Another instrument holds the ovary so that a thin needle can be placed in the follicle. The fluid that contains the egg is then drawn from the follicle. The patient is asleep with general anesthesia.

Figure 11.2 *(Pp. 183–184) Different techniques of egg retrieval. (Illustrations courtesy of IVF America.)*

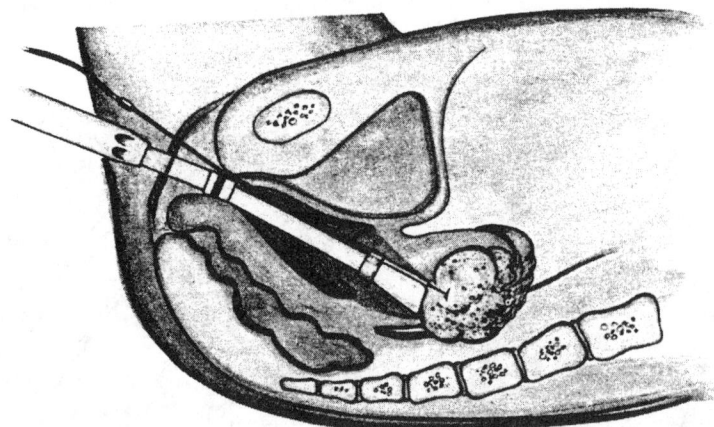

Nonsurgically (ultrasound-guided)
Ultrasound can be used to guide a thin needle through thin vaginal tissue to reach the follicle in the ovary. It allows a similar pregnancy rate as surgical retrieval.

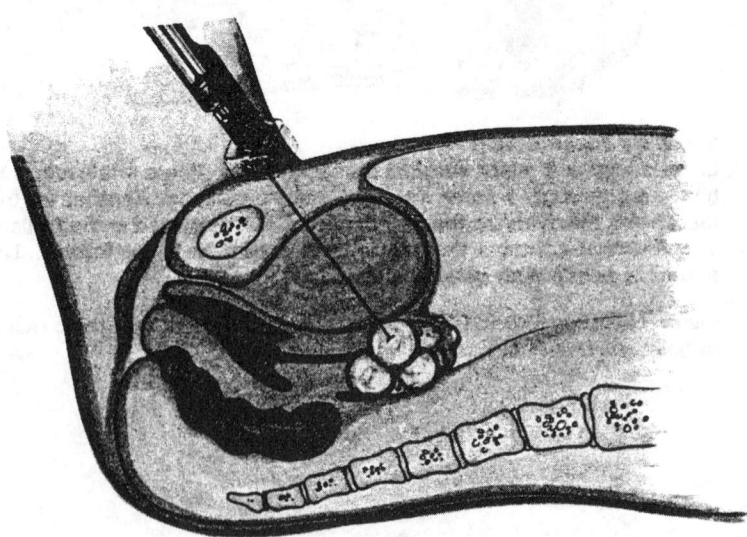

If the ovaries cannot be reached through the vagina, another approach can be used. Ultrasound can be used to guide a thin needle through the abdominal wall and bladder into the follicles.

nique, it is possible to take a sperm sample that would ordinarily have a very poor chance of fertilizing an egg in nature and use it more successfully with in vitro fertilization.

Fertilization and Embryo Transfer

This specially prepared sperm mixture is then added in precise amounts to each culture dish containing a single egg. The mixture sits in a closed space with a controlled environment—called an *incubator*—for about forty-eight hours, by which time fertilization should have occurred. After the egg is fertilized, it begins to divide. Somewhere between the two- and eight-cell stage of development, technicians remove the early embryo in its culture dish from the incubator. Then a technician attaches a long, very narrow plastic tube to a tiny syringe. By placing the free end of this tube in the culture dish next to the embryo and gently pulling the plunger back on the syringe, the technician can draw the embryo into the plastic tube. This procedure is repeated several times until ideally three or four of the embryos are withdrawn into one plastic tube (catheter).

The woman is then brought into a specially prepared room and lies in a normal pelvic examining position with a speculum in place. The physician carefully inserts the plastic tube containing the embryos through the cervical canal into the uterine cavity. By pushing down on the plunger of the syringe, the doctor expells the embryos from the plastic tube into the uterine cavity. The doctor then removes the catheter from the uterus and the patient is kept in the area for a short time and then sent home.

Over the next several weeks, blood samples are taken for human chorionic gonadotropin (HCG) levels; if an expected menstrual period does not occur, and the HCG levels are found to rise, pregnancy has occurred. If the patient has a positive pregnancy test and the HCG levels rise well, then we know that the pregnancy is surviving well. If the HCG levels rise only slightly for a short time and then rapidly fall, this is frequently called a *chemical pregnancy*. This means that the embryo died very soon after transfer occurred. If, on the other hand, the HCG levels continue to rise well, then eventually an ultrasound scan is done to locate the pregnancy to confirm that it is, in fact, within the uterus. Several weeks later, the ultrasound scan may be repeated to confirm that not only is the pregnancy in the uterus but that it is growing well. Once past these hurdles, the patient usually returns to the care of her obstetrician. Production of a pregnancy by in vitro fertilization does not make cesarean delivery necessary. Indeed, most women who have in vitro pregnancies deliver by normal vaginal delivery.

SOME IVF VARIATIONS

Although the scheme I have described is used in some programs, there are also certain variations. Some programs use clomiphene or Pergonal alone or certain combinations of clomiphene and Pergonal. At this time, it is difficult to say which, if any, of these stimulation techniques is superior to the rest.

Another variation is that the guidance of the needle used to retrieve the egg might be done by laparoscopy or by ultrasound. Some centers are currently using ultrasound to guide the placement of the needle through the abdomen into the follicles. This procedure was originally used in Denmark; centers throughout the world have gradually adopted it. The advantage of the use of ultrasound to follow the progress of the needle for egg retrieval is that it allows the recovery of eggs without the need to perform a laparoscopy, which is a surgical procedure.

Using ultrasound, a device, called a *transducer* is placed against the outside surface of your body. Looking something like a small flashlight, it emits high frequency sound waves that penetrate the body, bounce off organs, and return to the transducer. Here, the returning sound waves are converted into electrical impulses and conducted by way of a cable from the transducer to a device that looks like a small computer with a video screen. The electrical impulses are changed into an image that the operator can see on the ultrasound viewing screen. Thus, ultrasound visualization allows the physician to see a cross-sectional image of the human body at the point that the transducer touches its outer surface. This image can go through scar tissue and all surrounding structures. The result is that the physician can see an ovary that might be totally covered by other organs or adhesions and could not have been seen at all through laparoscopy.

In the vast majority of couples who attempt in vitro fertilization, the women have tubal scarring and damage, frequently from endometriosis, previous surgery, or ruptured appendices. Whatever the cause, women who attempt in vitro fertilization are as a group more apt to have very extensive abdominal scarring. Laparoscopy carries a greater inherent risk for a woman who has extensive scarring than for one with an unscarred abdomen. Scarring tends to displace the intestines and other structures in such a way that there is a greater possibility of inadvertent damage during the course of laparoscopic surgery. Furthermore once a laparoscope is inserted into the abdomen, the same scarring that has made it impossible for the Fallopian tube to function properly can cause intestines and adjacent structures to drape themselves over the surface of the ovaries so that it is difficult if not impossible to see them and accomplish egg retrieval.

Since ultrasound allows the physician to see through the abdominal wall and all areas of scarring, it is possible for him or her to use this technique to guide a needle into the abdomen through scar tissue and into a follicle. In this way, a doctor can retrieve eggs from women whose abdomens would make laparoscopy difficult, and it is just such women who tend to require in vitro fertilization most.

Since ultrasound-guided egg retrieval simply involves passing a needle—rather than a larger surgical instrument—into the body, general anaesthesia is not necessary, as it is for laparoscopy. Thus the risks associated with general anaesthesia are avoided. This method of retrieval must be considered one of the major advances in the evolution of in vitro fertilization.

There are several ways in which a doctor can introduce the needle into the abdominal cavity using ultrasound. Ovaries that have been stimulated in preparation for egg retrieval are significantly enlarged. The ovaries, which usually sit in back of the uterus, expand so that they are almost in contact with the wall of the vagina at their lower surface and project slightly to the side, almost to the level of the top of the uterus. A woman may be asked to drink enough water to allow her bladder to fill with urine and expand; then while she is lying on her back, a technician places the ultrasound transducer on the lower abdomen. The contents of the abdominal cavity appear on the video screen. This allows the physician to see a clear pathway from the abdominal wall through the bladder to the ovary. By passing a needle through the abdominal wall and the urinary bladder, it is possible to reach the ovary without penetrating any significant structure. The medical term for the urinary bladder is the "vesicle": this route of egg retrieval is called a *transabdominal transvesicle* ultrasound egg retrieval.

Another way of removing eggs by ultrasound is to pass the needle through the urethra, the tube through which urine is drained from the bladder. The doctor passes a long, thin needle through the urethra and through the back of the bladder into the ovary, again using an abdominal ultrasound transducer to produce a picture on a video screen for guidance. This technique is called *transurethral transvesicle* ultrasound retrieval.

The newest and probably the best route of retrieval is to pass the ultrasound transducer into the vagina. The transducer has a groove fitted into it to allow the long needle used for egg retrieval to be passed along its surface. The skin at the back of the vagina, separating the vagina from the abdominal cavity, is only about as thick as your earlobe. The doctor can insert the transducer deep within the vagina, up against the skin at the back of the vagina, where it can be only a fraction of an inch from the surface of the ovary. This small distance allows a clearer picture of the follicles and allows the needle to be passed more easily through a smaller amount of tissue into the follicles. Thus this technique is a rapid and more precise way of retrieving eggs. It is called *transvaginal* ultrasound-guided egg retrieval (Figure 11.2).

All three of these techniques can be carried out with intravenous sedation, avoiding the risks of general anaesthesia and its "hangover," as well as the general discomfort associated with laparoscopy. In most cases, a woman who has just undergone an ultrasound-guided egg retrieval can be up and moving about very quickly after the procedure. One of the most striking experiences I've had was trying to convince a woman who had had a transvaginal egg retrieval several hours earlier that perhaps it would not be a good idea to drive herself home alone. The only reason I insisted that her husband drive her home was because I was uncomfortable having a patient drive after any sedation. In my many years of infertility practice, I have never had a patient who wanted to drive herself home immediately after a laparoscopy.

SOME PROBLEMS AND SOLUTIONS

We must attempt to balance the fact that increasing the number of embryos transferred into the uterus at one time increases the probability of pregnancy with the fact that increasing the number of embryos also increases the probability of multiple births. Two embryos inserted at one time will give a couple a greater probability of pregnancy than one embryo. There is a similar increase as we put in three embryos rather than two. The probability of pregnancy increases less if we go to four embryos, and even less if we go to five. On the other hand, the probability of multiple births sharply increases as we go above four embryos transferred at one time. Thus, the point of diminishing returns appears to be somewhere above the level of three to four embryos. As we go above three to four embryos, the probability of pregnancy increases only slightly while the probability of multiple births increases significantly. Thus, the optimum number of embryos that should be transferred at any one time appears to be three to four.

If four embryos are transferred and the woman becomes pregnant, she has a 75% chance of delivering one baby, a 20% chance of twins, a 4% chance of triplets and a 1% chance of quadruplets. These percentages are estimates.

The greater the number of babies a woman carries in her uterus during a single pregnancy the greater the risks to both her and her babies. In a quadruplet pregnancy, the birth weight of each one of the four infants is smaller than that of each of twin babies. Low birth weight means that each baby is more vulnerable at its time of birth: it is more apt to develop brain damage as a result of bleeding in the brain as well as damage to nerve tissue. The delivery itself is more difficult. The obstetrician is faced with a tangle of arms, legs, and umbilical cords, so it becomes more difficult to effect a rapid delivery without cutting off the blood supply and therefore oxygen to any baby. Mothers carrying multiple babies tend to go into premature labor, thus delivering babies who would be small at term, even earlier, when survival is in significant doubt. A vaginal delivery of a quadruplet pregnancy would be very difficult, and most obstetricians choose to deliver these babies by cesarean section. Since the uterus is overstretched, like a balloon that has been inflated too many times, the uterus tends not to contract. When a uterus fails to contract, a postpartum hemorrhage can result. At times a hysterectomy has to be done in order to stop the bleeding. The woman also has a higher risk of high blood pressure and other medical complications during pregnancy. Very often a woman with a quadruplet pregnancy is put at absolute bedrest from the twelfth week of pregnancy until the time of delivery. For all of these reasons, a pregnancy with four or more fetuses is considered a high-risk situation and therefore undesirable.

If a couple had eight embryos resulting after a cycle of treatment, rather than transferring all eight into the uterus at one time and incurring the risks just discussed, it would be best to transfer four embryos and save the other four for a later time. This would actually give the couple a greater total chance of pregnancy while minimizing the risks of multiple births. We can "save" embryos by carefully preserving them in a special medium and freezing them in liquid nitrogen. The embryos can be thawed for use in a subsequent cycle. This procedure is called *cryopreservation*. About 75–90 percent of the embryos survive the freeze-thaw procedure, and those that do survive stand a good chance of producing pregnancy. If a couple achieves a pregnancy with the first set of embryos, and some remain in cryopreservation, this second group of embryos can be used to initiate a pregnancy at a later time without the woman having to go through an additional stimulation and retrieval.

Sperm preparation for in vitro fertilization selects the healthiest sperm from a population of cells released at any one time. A man who produces sperm of generally poor quality and cannot produce pregnancy under normal circumstances, can frequently produce a pregnancy by in vitro fertilization. The reason for this is that the sperm preparation in IVF selects the best sperm cells and IVF places these cells directly next to the egg, thus increasing the probability of fertilization. Although not all male factor problems are treatable by in vitro fertilization, there is clearly a population of men who would not be able to father a child in nature who will be successful through in vitro fertilization.

If both the man and the woman of a couple have severe fertility problems, in vitro fertilization may still be of value. There could be a situation where the woman has extensively scarred Fallopian tubes and the man produces sperm of extremely poor quality. In vitro fertilization can be used to collect the eggs. If the man's sperm sample is still not of sufficient quality to allow fertilization to take place, sperm from a donor can be used, with the couple's consent, to accomplish fertilization. Here the selection of a donor would be the same as in donor insemination (see discussion in Chapter 6).

If the woman is incapable of responding to the drugs given to induce ovulation, or if she has a genetic disease making it inappropriate to use one of her eggs, then an egg can be obtained from a donor. Here, an egg or eggs which have just been retrieved from another woman can be donated. For the sake of this discussion, let us consider the donor Woman A and the recipient couple, Couple B. An egg can be donated by Woman A and fertilized with the sperm of the man from Couple B. The resulting embryo would be put into the uterus of Woman B. This procedure has been done successfully and has resulted in the birth of several healthy babies. Egg donation has been done even in cases where Woman B does not have any functioning ovaries. In that case, the hormones that should have been provided by the ovary are given from the outside to help support the pregnancy during the early months. After the placenta begins to make the appropriate hormones, outside medication is no longer required.

If a couple is incapable of providing either sperm or eggs, then a donor embryo can be used. With the consent of both couples, your doctor can obtain an embryo from another couple undergoing in vitro fertilization and can transfer it into your uterus.

Thus in vitro fertilization can use donor sperm or donor eggs or a donor embryo.

GIFT

A variation of in vitro fertilization is a procedure described as the GIFT procedure. GIFT is an acronym for Gamete Intra-Fallopian Tube Transfer. In this technique, the woman is stimulated just as she would be for in vitro fertilization. The doctor performs a laparoscopy in a similar fashion; a technician prepares a sperm sample before the laparoscopy. After the doctor retrieves the eggs, he places them in a plastic tube with the sperm and reinserts them into the Fallopian tube at the time of the same laparoscopy. This procedure allows fertilization to take place within the Fallopian tube instead of a culture dish, as it does with in vitro fertilization. With GIFT, the woman must have at least one normal Fallopian tube.

Medical science believes that since fertilization takes place within the Fallopian tube, as it does in nature—rather than in a culture dish—pregnancy rates should be higher. Since it is a one-step procedure accomplished during a single laparoscopy, GIFT is considered a simpler procedure than in vitro fertilization.

The original pregnancy rates quoted for the GIFT procedure were better than 45 percent. Pregnancy rates of in vitro fertilization are generally expressed in two ways. One is the percentage of women who had eggs retrieved who finally became pregnant. Another expression of pregnancy rate is the percentage of women who had embryos transferred who became pregnant. At the time of the original presentation of the GIFT procedure, the pregnancy rates for in vitro fertilization were approximately 17 percent for retrieval and about 20 percent for transfer. At that time GIFT appeared to have a significantly higher rate than in vitro fertilization. Since then, IVF pregnancy rates have increased and GIFT pregnancy rates have gone down.

A study was done at Monash University in Australia, comparing pregnancy rates of in vitro fertilization and GIFT done in the same institution. Patients were randomly assigned to either IVF or GIFT. The pregnancy rates of the two procedures were identical. Thus the higher pregnancy rate for GIFT—one of the original stated advantages—may not be valid.

Another stated advantage of GIFT is its simplicity. However, with improvement in ultrasound technology, a rapid, more comfortable IVF egg retrieval can be accomplished by ultrasound rather than by surgical laparoscopy. GIFT, which at this time requires laparoscopy, appears to be more complex and invasive than IVF. Lastly, in vitro fertilization offers information that GIFT does not. If a couple fails to achieve a pregnancy after a GIFT cycle, the reason is not known. If a couple fails to achieve pregnancy after an IVF cycle, some information can be recouped. We know whether or not the eggs are fertilized; we know whether or not they divided; and whether or not the embryos looked good at the time of transfer. None of this information is available from GIFT.

WHEN TO CONSIDER IVF

In vitro fertilization and its variations are, in a sense, the court of last resort. They can offer the possibility of pregnancy to a woman who has extensively scarred Fallopian tubes or no tubes at all. They can be used when all other forms of treatment for infertility have been used without success.

IVF should be considered when a woman has had repeated ectopic pregnancies. After three ectopic pregnancies, the probability that a woman's next pregnancy will be ectopic is higher than the chance of its being uterine. Since the probability of an ectopic pregnancy is somewhere between 3 and 6 percent with in vitro fertilization, it is probably safer for a woman who has had several ectopic pregnancies to attempt her next pregnancy by in vitro fertilization.

There have been many advances in in vitro fertilization since the birth of Louise Brown. As we increase the number of eggs retrieved during a treatment cycle, we increase the number of embryos produced. The greater the number of embryos created, the greater the probability that a woman will become pregnant.

Though in vitro fertilization is indeed the court of last resort, it is a kind court. Whereas pregnancy rates were originally 17 percent for retrieval and 20 percent for transfer, they are now, in some programs, up to 29 percent for retrieval and 30 percent for transfer. The increased pregnancy rates are due to meticulous quality control and precision in every step of egg stimulation, retrieval, and transfer. We have reason to look forward to continued success and advances in this rapidly developing mode of treatment for infertility.

INDICATIONS FOR
IN VITRO FERTILIZATION

A woman and her doctor should consider in vitro fertilization if she is infertile from any of the following causes:

- Absence of both Fallopian tubes:
     Congenital
     Result of surgical removal
- Failed reconstructive tubal surgery.
- Severe tubal damage or extensive intraabdominal scarring where surgery would not be successful as judged by an experienced tubal surgeon.
- After a third ectopic pregnancy.
- Antisperm antibodies—man's and/or woman's—unresponsive to medical treatment.
- Low sperm count unresponsive to conventional treatment.
- Endometriosis:—
     When infertility persists in spite of adequate surgery and/or drug treatment. (IVF has no effect on endometriosis itself.)
- Infertility of undetermined origin.
- All failed adequate infertility therapies.

I have referred to IVF as "the court of last resort," but perhaps this term conveys the wrong feeling. Perhaps a better term is "another chance." IVF is another opportunity to produce a child when other efforts have been unsuccessful, to possibly succeed in the fulfillment of an infertile couple's dream.

CHAPTER 12

High Tech and Newer Treatment

WE ARE living at a time when engineering, physics, and general technology are becoming married to medical therapy. The result is a rapid evolution in the technical means available to treat medical problems. This technology uses magnification, laser energy, and ultrasound to allow the physician to accomplish things unheard of five to ten years ago.

MICROSURGERY

Scarring around the Fallopian tubes and/or ovaries is a primary cause of infertility in 30 percent of infertile couples. The only way to offer these couples a chance to achieve a pregnancy is either to surgically correct any structural problems involving the Fallopian tubes or to bypasss the whole circuit through in vitro fertilization (See Chapter 11).

Successful reconstructive surgery, unlike in vitro fertilization, allows a couple to achieve pregnancy in the privacy of their own home without the continued involvement of technology and drug treatment, so there is a certain basic desirability of surgery as a technique to restore fertility. As in vitro fertilization evolves, however, a point may come when it may be the more efficient technique.

In order for the Fallopian tubes to function properly, they must be able to move easily to pick up any eggs released from the surface of the ovary. Sometimes bands of connective tissue—forming sheets or strands—will form. These connections are known as adhesions and may be the result of any process that irritates the tissue within the abdominal cavity. A low-grade pelvic infection that may be so minimal as to be without any symptoms can be just such an irritating adhesion-producing process. An ovarian cyst that ruptures and releases an irritating fluid can produce an inflammation of neighboring tissues and bands of adhesions, another possible source of pelvic scar tissue formation. The generation of adhesions appears to be part of the protective process the body uses to wall off irritation and prevent it from spreading throughout the abdominal cavity. In a certain sense, this is of tremendous survival value to the individual, because it prevents the spread of potentially damaging disease. For that reason many women develop pelvic adhesions very easily. On the other hand, such scar tissue formation may hamper tubal movement and therefore tubal functioning. The result may be infertility.

Another possibility may be that the Fallopian tube, rather than ending in an open structure that can pick up an egg, is sealed at its outer end (Figure 12.1). The result is that the tube, instead of looking very much like a long trumpet with the fimbria at its wider end, looks like a long balloon with the tube sealed at the portion closest to the ovary. In the same way the Fallopian tube may be blocked in the midportion, and the result here, too, is infertility.

For many years, surgeons have been restoring the structure of the Fallopian tube, cutting away scar tissue and removing obstructions. But with conventional surgery the results in terms of pregnancy have been dismal. Tubes closed up again, and scar tissue that was removed frequently formed again and sometimes actually worsened. The result was a markedly low pregnancy rate. It became clear that new techniques had to be develped.

Surgeons realized that tubal infertility surgery required very precise reconstruction. It was not good enough to just cut away an obstructed portion of the tube, suture the two ends back together again, and hope that they would heal in a continuous, unobstructed state. Somehow, surgeons had to see the lining and

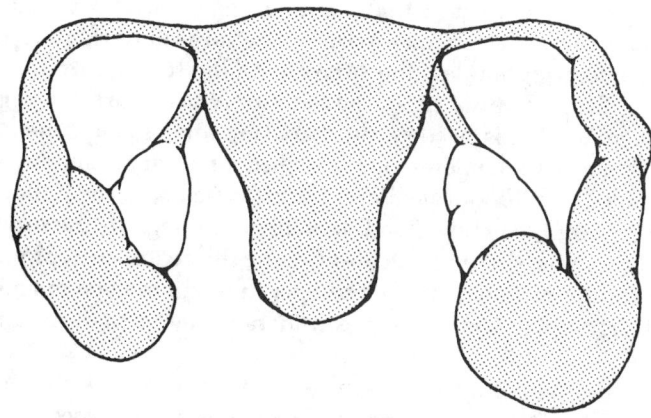

Figure 12.1 *Hydrosalpinx. Both tubes are closed and enlarged into two thin-walled, saclike structures. These tubes are unable to pick up an egg.*

the muscle layer of the tube as separate structures and reconstruct these very thin layers. When attempting to rejoin two ends of a severed tube, the surgeon must perfectly align the channels within the tube. The surgeon must then suture thin muscle layers together and cover the whole tube with a smooth, flawless surface, allowing no bleeding or oozing from the area of surgical repair. It became clear that seeing the structures with the naked eye was not enough: some form of magnification was necessary. The sutures used in these reconstructions had to be of finer materials, sometimes going to diameters approaching that of a human hair and even smaller. It was found that the smaller the diameter of the suture, the less it irritated the tissue in which it lay. Thus, surgeons began to see the need for microsurgery.

The use of very fine sutures to deal with small structures requires the use of magnification. In order to see these tiny structures, surgeons sometimes use loupes and at other times microscopes. An operating loupe looks very much like a small black eyepiece used by jewelers to examine watches and gems.

The operating loupe is actually a set of small telescopes attached to a pair of eyeglass frames worn by the surgeon during surgery. Using operating loupes, the surgeon is able to magnify the operating field up to six times. Sometimes, when a greater degree of magnification is needed, an operating microscope is helpful. This is an actual microscope attached to a large column and suspended over the surgical area. It is focused onto the Fallopian tube, or other structures, and, by looking through it, the surgeon is able to gain the magnification he or she requires to properly perform the reconstruction. The operating microscope magnifies the image up to forty times, considerably more than a pair of loupes.

The term *microsurgery* means surgery performed with the aid of magnification, either a loupe or an operating microscope. The term implies a greater order of surgical precision, using very fine, nonirritating sutures, and gentle tissue handling. Microsurgery has taught surgeons that the key to the most successful outcome is handling tissue carefully.

With ordinary surgical technique, surgeons used to blot excess blood from the operative field using an absorbent gauzelike material formed into sheets, called laparotomy pads. When observing these same areas under a microscope, surgeons suddenly became aware of the fact that what had been a routine technique for removing blood actually traumatizes the underlying tissue. In some cases this trauma results in scar tissue formation. Thus, the use of a microscope has made surgeons more attentive to the sensitivity and vulnerability of normal tissue, making them treat the structures being reconstructed with greater respect and gentleness. New techniques have evolved that will allow the removal of blood and clot without damage to the underlying structures. Microsurgery also has made it apparent that if tissue is exposed to the air and allowed to dry out, the surfaces become damaged, which leads to more scar tissue formation. So a microsurgeon operates under a constantly moistened or "wet" operating field. Even the composition of the fluid that is used to moisten the tissue becomes important. Special salt solutions are used to protect the tissues.

Basically, microsurgery is as much a philosophy as it is a set of surgical techniques. It is a surgical approach with meticulous attention to detail. It includes a devout respect for tissue integrity and dictates handling the tissue most delicately.

We can make a distinction between microsurgical technique and actual microsurgery. Microsurgical technique is the above emphasis on detail. Actual microsurgery is all of the above plus the use of magnification. There are times when magnification is not appropriate, such as for the removal of a large fibroid from a uterus or for a uterine reconstruction. Even when the structure being operated on is as large as a baseball, the general philosophy of microsurgery can still be used and is very beneficial.

Microsurgical technique introduces certain problems that are not of consequence in ordinary surgery. Every person has a normal physiological movement of his or her hands. This movement, frequently referred to as tremor, varies from individual to individual and in the same individual under different circumstances. A surgeon's tremor may not be sufficient to be noticeable under normal circumstances, but might be disruptive to the surgeon working under a microscope. Because tremor may hamper precise movement such as dissecting or suturing, the microsurgeon must try to minimize it by avoiding alcohol, caffeine, nicotine, severe muscular exertion, and anxiety.

Microsurgical instruments must have very fine, sharp tips on them so that they can grab minute structures that are seen under the microscope. Very special care is needed to protect these delicate instruments. In order to suture these tiny structures, small needles with very narrow diameter suture material are used. The sutures are frequently made of nylon, Dexon, or Vicryl. These materials produce very little irritation of the tissue in which they are placed.

Thus microsurgery, as a technique even without a microscope, influences the suture material, the needle selection, the shape and the care of the instruments, and the very way the microsurgeon lives his or her life. The results of all of this effort are very gratifying.

Let us examine one of several kinds of infertility operations to see how microsurgery has changed the results. If a woman has had a sterilization procedure, usually a part of the middle of the

Fallopian tube was removed, interrupting the continuity of the tube: it is not a continuous channel that will allow an egg to be conducted from the ovary to the uterus. After this surgery, called a tubal ligation, the egg remains at the outer portion of the tube and the sperm at the uterine side of the tube. Thus the egg and the sperm can never meet, and the result is a form of permanent contraception. If you want to reverse this procedure, the two portions must be rejoined. When the tubes are reconnected using regular surgical techniques, the pregnancy rates vary between 15 and 20 percent. When microsurgical techniques are used with an operating microscope, the pregnancy rates vary between 70 and 80 percent. Thus, a tremendous increase in the pregnancy rate occurs with meticulous care of the tissue and finer suturing techniques.

For this operation, you go under anesthesia in an operating room, and the surgeon makes an incision in your abdomen. The microsurgeon looks for your tubes and finds the area on each tube that had been cut away to produce tubal obstruction and therefore a tubal ligation. Using a very fine pair of scissors, the surgeon cuts away the obstructed portion of the tube and begins the procedure of anastomosing (rejoining) the healthy tube sections (Figure 12.2). Using an operating microscope, the surgeon can see the tube segments on each side of the uterus. Starting first on the one side, the surgeon places a series of very thin sutures around the circumference of the tube in the muscle, just outside of the inner channel of the tube, reestablishing the continuity of the channel within the tube. Then the surgeon places a second layer of sutures around the outside "plastic wrap-like" membrane of the Fallopian tube—called peritoneum—that creates a smooth, slippery covering over the operative site. To the naked eye it seems as though no damage or surgery had been done in this area. The surgeon does this to both Fallopian tubes, and then injects dye inside the uterus and watches it fill and spill out of both tubes, demonstrating that the anastomosis was successful on both sides. The surgery is usually tolerated very well, and you can go home in less than a week.

Microsurgical technique can also be used to remove scar tissue from around the reproductive structures. While you are under

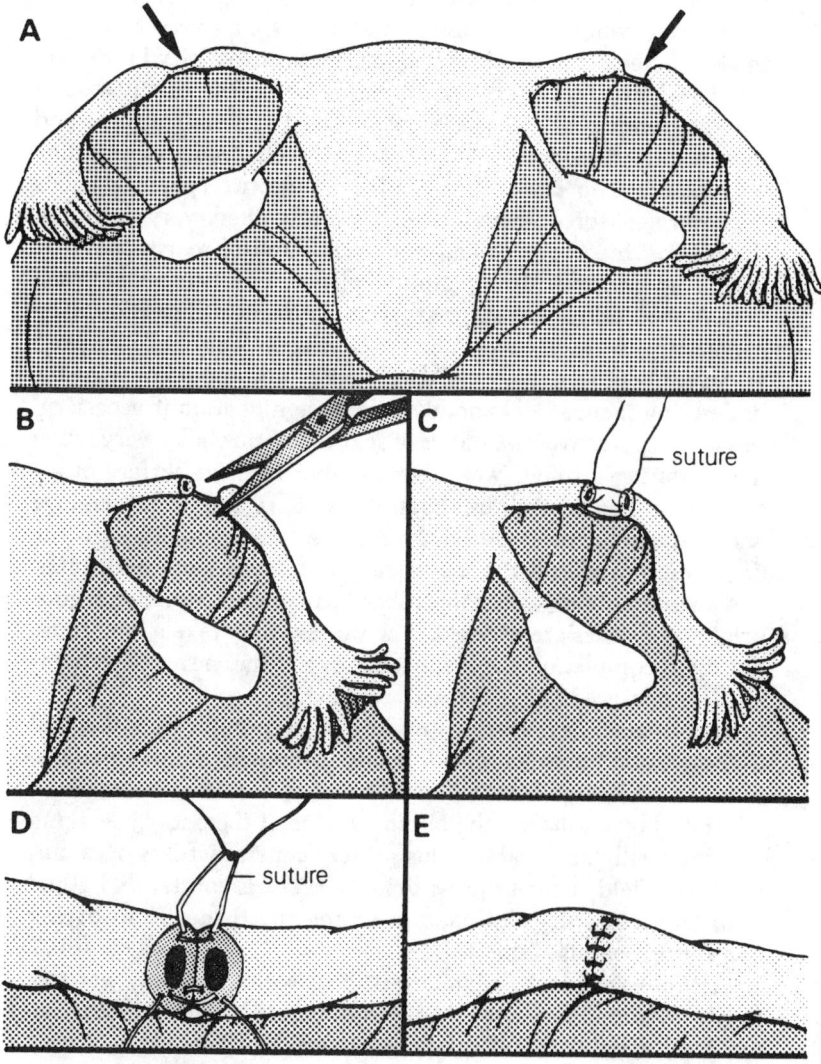

Figure 12.2 *Technique of reversal of a tubal ligation. The obstructed segment of each tube is cut out and the tube segments sewn back together (anastomosis).*

general anesthesia, the surgeon makes an incision in your abdomen exposing the uterus and tubes. The surgeon notes that both tubes are covered with dense adhesions, looking very much like thick cobwebs. But unlike cobwebs, these sheets of whitish material feel like thin plastic or thread. The doctor briefly studies the relationship of the adhesions to the tubes and ovaries and then begins dissection. Using a needle-tip electrode—a very fine wire attached to a source of controlled electric current—and a microsurgical forcep with a carefully maintained, very sharp tip, the microsurgeon grasps and cuts each band of scar tissue. The needle-tip electrode, using minimal electric current, can cut each area of scar tissue, creating an almost bloodless dissection. The needle-tip electrode's action is very similar to that of a laser; both are capable of removing scar tissue with minimal damage to the underlying tissue. Occasionally using magnification if necessary, the surgeon removes the bands of scar tissue carefully, very much like stripping a spider web fiber by fiber from its surface of attachment. The careful dissection is necessary to prevent damage and trauma to the underlying tissue. At the completion of the dissection—when all the scar tissue is removed from both tubes and ovaries—once again the tubes, with intact functional fimbria, and ovaries are exposed. The surgery may take a long time, but upon completion the tissue looks as if it had never been damaged or operated on.

In both cases the surgery is usually done through what is called a Pfannenstiel incision. This is a side-to-side abdominal incision, sometimes referred to as a "bikini incision" because it is made at or a bit above or below the pubic hairline of the patient, making it cosmetically acceptable. This surgery generally takes place under a wet field, which means that the tissue is constantly bathed with a special salt solution, preventing the tissues from drying out and becoming damaged.

At times the results of microsurgical technique may not improve the pregnancy rate. Sometimes it just means that scar tissue production is reduced. This is a very significant step. Every time the abdomen is opened, the contents of the abdominal cavity are disturbed and irritated, increasing the possibility of scar tissue production. The use of heavy suture and the handling of tissue within the abdomen, increase the chances of scar tissue formation as well. Since all of these things are part and parcel in abdominal surgery, it is surprising that all such surgery does not result in a great amount of scar tissue being produced. Scar tissue can cause chronic pelvic pain, intestinal obstruction, and infertility. Microsurgical techniques, even without magnification, produce less of an insult to the abdominal organs and therefore reduce the chances of scar tissue and adhesion formation.

These are not the only surgical procedures to be carried out by microsurgery. Other procedures include a salpingostomy, which is opening up an obstructed fimbrial portion of the tube. There is a certain sense in which all abdominal surgical procedures, whether performed on a woman of reproductive age or not, or even on a man, should be considered appropriate for microsurgical technique. After all, there should be no reason why anyone should have a greater amount of surgical tissue trauma than is necessary. Microsurgery is not a cure-all. Tubes can still close after surgery and adhesions may still reform, but microsurgery and microsurgical technique shift the odds in favor of success.

Microsurgery is not the answer to all structural infertility problems. But it does take a giant step forward toward allowing more careful and successful reconstruction for everyone who requires such surgery. It is a significant improvement over previous surgical techniques and is a basis on which ideal reconstructions of the future can build.

LASERS

The surgeon reconstructs tissue by cutting into the tissue surfaces. Until very recently, this involved the use of a sharp instrument called a scalpel. It is used to slice across the surface being cut. In order to do this, pressure is exerted on the scalpel, the tissue is compressed and its surface distorted. If the tissue could somehow be cut with energy rather than mechanical force, the sculpturing of the tissue surface could be carried out more accurately. Tissues could be cut without distorting the surfaces, and a more perfect rendering of the desired forms could be made.

In the 1960s it was found that electrical energy could be used toward this end. Using a small electrode attached to a current generator, electrical energy can be concentrated into a tiny surface of tremendous density. This results in the vaporization of cells at the point of contact between the tissue and the electrode. Very often a bleeding blood vessel can be closed with the same electrode. This technique, called electrosurgery, allows the surgeon to cut tissues without any major compression or distortion of the tissue surface, with minimal tissue trauma and bleeding.

Another way of accomplishing the same thing is by using light energy. If light is focused in a particular way, with all of the wave forms highly concentrated and in phase, the energy can also vaporize tissue. This is generally the principle of the laser. The word "laser" is actually an abbreviation for "light amplification by stimulated emission of radiation." By selecting lasers, of different light sources, we can affect tissue in different ways.

In gynecology, three major types of lasers are used. These are: the carbon dioxide laser, the YAG laser, and the argon laser. The carbon dioxide laser can cut tissue very easily and can close off small blood vessels. Cutting tissue by use of a carbon dioxide laser allows making an incision with minimal bleeding. However, if a blood vessel of significant size is cut, bleeding still occurs. So the claims of bloodless surgery using carbon dioxide lasers are frequently inaccurate and overstated. The amount of surrounding tissue damage that occurs around an incision caused by the carbon dioxide laser usually is minimal. Like electrical surgery or conventional surgery with a scalpel, the important factor here is the amount of trauma that is produced to surrounding tissue. If care is taken to keep the power of the carbon dioxide laser to a minimum, the amount of damage is also minimized. The point is that the same care that is carried out in conventional surgery must be applied to carbon dioxide laser surgery. Carbon dioxide laser surgery may still produce scarring and it is not true that the carbon dioxide laser produces surgery without any scarring of the incision.

The YAG and argon lasers are capable of producing greater amounts of coagulation of bleeding blood vessels than the carbon dioxide laser. These lasers do not cut quite as well as the carbon dioxide laser but can seal blood vessels, creating incisions that are truly potentially bloodless. However, the amount of surrounding tissue damage with the YAG and argon lasers is potentially greater than that of the carbon dioxide laser.

Technology in each one of these laser areas is evolving very rapidly. The result is that the positive and negative sides to the use of each of the lasers are being refined and removed, respectively. Over the last several years, engineers have been able to decrease the amount of surrounding tissue damage associated with the YAG laser by changing its delivery system. The carbon dioxide laser has an improved delivery system, too. In the very near future, the differences among these lasers will probably diminish.

The main advantage of the laser is that it can be delivered into the body through fibers or small telescopes. The result is that some of the surgical procedures that used to require full abdominal surgery can now be performed by operative laparoscopy and hysteroscopy. Patients can go home much sooner and their surgical outcome is the same or perhaps even better than in full abdominal surgery. It remains to be demonstrated which surgical procedures are best performed by laser endoscopy and which by abdominal surgery. It also remains to be demonstrated that lasers can accomplish anything more than careful use of electrical instruments. Both lasers and electrical instruments have the potential of damaging surrounding tissue. Each one can produce inadvertent damage to bowel, bladder, uterus, blood vessels, and other surrounding structures. The magic bullet that can destroy only undesired scar tissue and endometriosis—leaving normal tissue intact and undamaged—unfortunately has not yet been found.

ULTRASOUND

Using telescopes inserted through the human body, surgeons are frequently able to see obscure structures. The hysteroscope is used to see the inside of the uterine cavity, and the laparoscope can be used to allow the surgeon to look inside the abdomen. These are surgical procedures requiring insertion of an instrument into the human body. In this sense they are described as being invasive. It would be helpful to find a way to look into a human body without actually inserting a device into the body itself; that is, using noninvasive techniques. X-rays allow the observer to differentiate bony tissue from soft tissues, but it is frequently difficult to tell one kind of soft tissue structure from another. X-rays are unable to see the uterus and ovaries. In other words, these structures are entirely invisible using X-rays.

But sound waves that are emitted from a small device called a transducer, can be sent through the human body. The sound waves will bounce off soft tissue structures and return to the transducer. These signals can be reconstructed into visual images and can be used to "see" soft tissue structure in ultrasound. Using ultrasound technology, the physician is able to see the Fallopian tube, ovary, uterus, and so on. The problem is that the resolution of the ultrasound picture is not good enough to clearly see scar tissue bands and to differentiate these structures from tubes and ovaries. Until relatively recently ultrasound was very helpful in describing larger soft tissue structure but not very good at describing fine variations in the shape of small structures. But as the ability of ultrasound devices to generate more precise images has improved and the general technology has changed, the usefulness of ultrasound has increased. Today, by placing an ultrasound transducer on the abdomen or even within the vagina, it is possible to diagnose the presence of an embryo within the uterine cavity. It is frequently possible to locate an embryo that is abnormally placed outside the uterine cavity by using ultrasound. Ultrasound techniques can be used to help measure and count the number of follicles in an ovary during Pergonal stimulation or during in vitro fertilization treatment. Abdominal and/or vaginal transducers can be used to guide the collection of eggs for in vitro fertilization. (See Chapter 11.)

GnRH ANALOGUES

Estrogen is produced by the ovary under stimulation by FSH and LH from the pituitary gland. The pituitary, in turn, is stimulated by a protein from the hypothalamus called GnRH, (gonadotropin-releasing hormone). GnRH is released in a pulsing fashion, with releases occurring approximately six minutes out of every ninety minutes on a regular basis. If this signal is changed so that GnRH is released in a longer or more frequent fashion, FSH and LH are no longer produced by the pituitary. Without FSH and LH, the ovary ceases to function and estrogen levels fall. This is the principle behind therapy using GnRH analogues.

GnRH analogue is a substance that behaves very much like GnRH but has a slight change in structure allowing it to behave slightly differently. If the drug behaves like GnRH but is longer acting, it is called a long-acting analogue. When such analogues are created, they behave like a continuous signal of GnRH occurring longer than six minutes out of every ninety minutes. The result is that long-acting analogues produce a drop in FSH and LH production. This drop is followed by a fall in estrogen levels. Structures that are causing problems and that rely on estrogen can best be treated with long-acting GnRH analogues. Endometriosis implants require estrogen to survive. Giving patients with endometriosis GnRH analogues has been found to be very successful therapy. Implants shrivel, and there are far fewer side effects than with most other forms of current therapy.

Benign tumors of the uterus called leiomyomata—more commonly referred to as fibroids—also require estrogen for their survival. Giving patients GnRH analogues also results in a dramatic reduction of uterine fibroids. We can take a large fibroid that might require radical surgery and reduce it to a very small size by administering a GnRH analogue. These analogues can be delivered in many different ways; one form is by nasal spray, another is by injection. After GnRH therapy ends, the structures frequently begin to enlarge, sometimes in as little as six months. When a fibroid is preventing pregnancy, then the suppression of its growth by GnRH analogue may provide enough opportunity to allow a pregnancy to occur. Even if this opportunity lasts only six months, it may be sufficient. Another possibility is that GnRH therapy may convert a difficult surgical procedure into a simpler one so that surgery can be carried out with greater probability of preserving the integrity of the uterus. The result is that in the near-future GnRH treatment may allow many women who now require surgical treatment for both endometriosis and/or fibroids to avoid surgery entirely. In women who still require surgery it will take the case from a difficult procedure to a much simpler one.

A shorter-acting GnRH analogue can be administered to induce ovulation. This may be successful in stimulating ovulation in women who do not respond well to either clomiphene or Pergonal.

Investigators have recently experimented with the combined administration of a long-acting GnRH analogue and Pergonal. This combination seems to result in better stimulation of ovulation in anovultory women who do not respond well to Pergonal alone. The same drug combination is also useful in *in vitro* fertilization to produce a larger number and/or better-quality follicles and eggs in women who do not respond well to the usual stimulation protocols. In other words, many women who have a variety of ovulatory problems appear to be treatable using the combination of a long-acting GnRH analogue and Pergonal.

CHORIONIC VILLUS SAMPLING

With the mother's increasing age, the probability of fetal abnormality increases. Since the point is not simply to achieve a pregnancy but to deliver a healthy child, the detection of fetal abnormalities becomes an important form of evaluation, particularly if the mother is over the age of thirty-five. If an abnormality is found, the couple may elect to terminate the pregnancy. If the couple elects to allow the pregnancy to continue, that decision will have been based on knowledge, and, if necessary, preparations for special care immediately after delivery can be made well in advance.

Amniocentesis has been the classic way of evaluating the genetic composition of an unborn child. In this procedure your doctor inserts a needle through your abdominal wall and uterus into the amniotic fluid, the liquid in which the fetus floats. The amniotic fluid contains cells and body chemicals from the fetus. By sampling this fluid, these cells can be collected and studied for their genetic composition. Thus, a genetic evaluation of the unborn child is possible. This procedure is usually done between the fourteenth and sixteenth weeks of pregnancy, and it takes several weeks for the results of the studies to return. This means that if the pregnancy will be terminated, it must be done around the eighteenth week. The period of time that a couple must wait for the results and the trauma of terminating the pregnancy this late in its development can make the amniocentesis a very difficult procedure.

Recently, a new method called *chorionic villus sampling*, or CVS, has been introduced. It is usually done before the tenth week of pregnancy, and the results come back in one to five days. Thus, if a pregnancy is to be terminated, the procedure can be done more easily and the period of time that a couple must experience the stress of waiting for the results is significantly shortened.

To perform this procedure, the physician inserts a narrow plastic tube through the vagina and cervix, into the very edge of the uterine cavity. Here, under ultrasound guidance, a small piece of tissue from the placental area—representing an area of fetal cells—is withdrawn into the tube and the doctor removes the tube from the uterus. The tissue is sent to the laboratory where genetic studies are performed.

Following the procedure, you may stain for several hours or days. The main concern is that the miscarriage rate following this procedure may be higher than that following conventional amniocentesis. Miscarriage rate has been estimated to be approximately 2 percent, but some investigators have quoted numbers considerably higher.

One of the potential benefits is that CVS allows the rapid evaluation of a pregnancy in progress at a time when the pregnancy can easily be terminated. Its disadvantages include the possible higher risk of fetal loss. There appears little doubt that in the near future the technique of CVS will improve and its widespread use will become far more extensive. For the moment most institutions consider it experimental.

SURROGATE MOTHERHOOD

A woman who is unable to carry her own pregnancy can retain another woman to do it for her. This second woman is identified as a *surrogate mother*. The surrogate can become pregnant by having a doctor perform artificial insemination using the sperm of the man of the first couple. She may also become pregnant by having a doctor transfer an embryo into her that is the product of the sperm of the man and the egg of the woman of the couple who have retained the surrogate. In this sense, the surrogate is used as a substitute to bear the child for another woman. The arrangement is set down in a contract, but the only way to know how binding this legal document is, is to have it tested in court. Contracts between the donor parents and surrogate mothers are sophisticated and will continue to evolve. However, it is uncertain what provisions of such contracts are feasible. Not all circumstances are foreseeable, and it would be naive to hope for a contract that could truly cover all eventualities. Laws governing adoption fall under the jurisdiction of state government, so it is anticipated that clauses tied to surrogacy arrangements, its related issues, and their resolution would be handled by state, rather than federal courts.

Surrogacy at this time represents a vast area of uncharted waters and any couple considering entering into such an agreement should do so with great caution, if at all.

This has been a brief look at the newest developments in reproductive medicine—the possible and the almost possible. Some of the procedures in this chapter, as well as earlier chapters, are not in general use and are still considered somewhat experimental. The possibilities for the future are exciting and many. The results of current research will mean conception for those couples who are untreatable today. At this moment there is no question in my mind that the advances outlined in this chapter will be in general use soon and that more advances are coming. The question is only, "How soon?" The only thing more exciting than imagining what the future will bring is working in an area of medical research that will actually produce those advances, and being able to tell a couple once thought to be untreatable, "Congratulations, the pregnancy test is positive. You're pregnant!"

CHAPTER 13

Pregnancy Over Thirty-five

WE ARE entering a time in which there will be a major increase in the number of births to women in their mid-thirties and beyond. This, in part, reflects changes in our society, allowing and encouraging women to pursue careers and to delay childbearing. This also reflects the growing up of the baby boomers who were born in the middle of this century. The highest number of births ever recorded in the United States occurred between 1947 and 1965. Women born at the early part of this time reached their thirty-fifth birthdays in the early 1980s, while those born around 1965 will be reaching thirty-five around the year 2000. During this twenty-year period, there will be more women in the later childbearing years than at any time in our history. The result is that a great deal of attention must be directed toward ferreting out, addressing, and treating reproductive problems associated with increased maternal age. In general, after the age of thirty-five, fertility rates decrease, complications to the mother during pregnancy increase, and fetal complication rates rise. It becomes important to address each one of these areas independently.

After age thirty-five, there appears to be an increasing frequency of ovulatory abnormality. As a woman approaches age forty, the probability of irregular ovulation and of progesterone deficiencies when ovulation does occur increases. After age forty, even though ovulation may occur, the endometrium, the lining of the uterus, does not seem to respond appropriately. Your doctor can treat ovulatory abnormalities that result from your age with any of the usual drugs used to treat ovulation problems (See Chapter 6). Problems of the poorly responding endometrium may or may not be treatable. You and your doctor have to make judgments as part of your individual evaluation. The bottom line is that though ovulatory abnormality is a problem, it is usually approachable but demands a greater degree of attention if you are over thirty-five.

Older women who do become pregnant, particularly those who are over the age of forty, have a higher risk of maternal complications. There is a higher incidence of elevated blood pressure during pregnancy, which is associated with impaired growth of the fetus and an increased risk of miscarriage. Another blood pressure-related problem is called preeclampsia. This is a form of elevated blood pressure that is associated only with pregnancy. If left untreated, it can lead to convulsions and significant damage to both mother and unborn child. On the other hand, elevated blood pressure associated with pregnancy, whether due to simple hypertension or preeclampsia, is treatable.

Diabetes may appear during pregnancy, and its probability increases with maternal age. Diabetes during pregnancy affects the quality of the pregnancy and the survival of the fetus. Therefore, it becomes critical that each woman over the age of thirty-five be screened for diabetes during pregnancy. If found, diabetes should be tightly controlled.

Labors of women who are over the age of thirty-five progress less well and so cesarean section rate increases directly with an increase in maternal age. The placenta may be improperly positioned and this condition, too, requires greater attention during labor and delivery.

Lastly, there is increased risk to the fetus in pregnancies over the age of thirty-five, because there is a greater chance of genetic abnormalities. The chances increase year by year, increase markedly after the age of thirty-five, and increase at a far greater rate after the age of forty. (See Table 13.1.) Thus it becomes very important to evaluate the genetic composition of your fetus. The important point in achieving pregnancy is not simply getting a positive pregnancy test but having a normal child, creating a new, healthy human being who will be a contribution to your family and society. It is for this reason that we strongly encourage women over thirty-five to obtain a genetic evaluation of their pregnancies. This can include amniocentesis or chorionic villus sampling.

There is also an increased risk of pregnancy loss, premature delivery, stillbirth, and death of a baby following delivery that can be related in some way to increasing maternal age.

We know from information collected from in vitro fertilization studies that it is harder to stimulate women over forty to mature several eggs at the same time. The same drug stimulation that works well in women in their late thirties will be less apt to work at age forty and forty-one. When the eggs are finally obtained, they appear to be just as fertilizable as eggs obtained from younger women, but when the embryos are produced and transferred into the uterus, their rate of survival is reduced. From this information, it seems likely that some of the reproductive problems seen in women in their later childbearing years are due to the response of the follicle and the ovary to the woman's pituitary stimulation. Some of the problems are associated with the environment the uterus provides for the developing embryo; this environment appears to be markedly diminished in quality after the age of forty.

EVALUATION AND TREATMENT

Thus, there are certain factors in reproduction at an older age that can be controlled and watched, and others that are beyond our control. Infertility over thirty-five that may be due to ovulatory abnormalities and progesterone dysfunctions can be treated in the same way as in a younger woman. Once a woman over the age of thirty-five becomes pregnant, it becomes important to evaluate the pregnancy to be sure of its genetic composition. If the studies are abnormal, serious consideration of termination of the pregnancy should be made. This does not mean that all genetically abnormal pregnancies need to be terminated. The decision can be made by the couple based on knowledge, and if necessary, preparations for special care immediately after delivery can be made well in advance.

There are two general ways of obtaining genetic information about an ongoing pregnancy. The classical way is to perform an amniocentesis. While in the uterus, the fetus floats in a waterlike environment called amniotic fluid, shedding cells and body chemicals into this liquid world. By inserting a long needle through the abdominal wall, into the uterus, and into the amniotic fluid, a doctor can withdraw some of this material and perform tests. This sampling procedure is called amniocentesis and is usually done between the fourteenth and sixteenth weeks of pregnancy. The cells removed from the amniotic fluid can be cultured to study their genetic composition. Using this, Down syndrome, previously known as mongolism, as well as other genetic diseases, can be diagnosed well before birth. The chemical composition of the fluid can also be analyzed to diagnose certain other fetal abnormalities that are not related to genetic problems. Some abnormalities associated with the formation of the central nervous system are not a result of genetic causes but may still be critical in the development of the baby. Doing specialized chemical studies on the amniotic fluid can sometimes allow the diagnosis of such problems relatively early in pregnancy.

Another way of evaluating the genetic material of a pregnancy is to perform a *chorionic villus biopsy*. This procedure is also called a chorionic villus sampling, abbreviated CVS. In this procedure a doctor inserts a small plastic tube into the edge of the uterine cavity through the cervix and using ultrasound guidance, removes a small amount of tissue from the placenta. This tissue is cultured and studies are performed to evaluate the genetic information of the fetus. The advantage of CVS over amniocentesis is that it can provide information at a much earlier time in pregnancy, usually at about six to eight weeks, as opposed to the fourteen–sixteen weeks needed for the amniocentesis. On the other hand, chorionic villus sampling does not provide all the biochemical information that amniocentesis can provide. Further development in the technology of CVS will probably bring it up to the level of amniocentesis in the very near future.

When a woman thirty-five or older becomes pregnant, it is important that she receive close medical followup. Her doctor should screen her for diabetes and hypertensive diseases of pregnancy. Genetic evaluation of the fetus should be carried out and, if a problem is discovered, she and her partner may want to consider ending the pregnancy to prevent the birth of an abnormal child. Using such an approach, the risk of pregnancy to a mother over the age of thirty-five can be sharply reduced.

An important warning to remember is that if you are thirty-five or older and fail to conceive after six months of regular unprotected intercourse instead of the usual twelve months, you and your partner should begin an infertility evaluation.

Following the principles set out in this chapter a woman of age thirty-five or above can maximize her chances of pregnancy.

Table 13:1: Relationship of Maternal Age to Chromosomol Abnormalities

Estimated Rates at Time of Expected Live Birth

Maternal Age	Down's Syndrome	All Chromosomal Abnormalities
25	1/1250	1/500
30	1/950	1/400
31	1/900	1/400
32	1/800	1/300
33	1/600	1/275
34	1/500	1/250
35	1/400	1/175
36	1/300	1/150
37	1/225	1/125
38	1/175	1/100
39	1/125	1/75
40	1/100	1/60
41	1/80	1/50
42	1/60	1/40
43	1/50	1/30
44	1/40	1/25
45	1/30	1/20
46	1/25	1/15
47	1/20	1/10
48	1/15	1/10
49	1/10	1/5

CHAPTER 14
Closing Thoughts

THE TITLE of this chapter is "closing thoughts," rather than "final thoughts." At this point, I want to present some extraneous ideas that do not fit easily into any of the categories I've discussed thus far. They are not the final thoughts on the subject of fertility. In fact, if there is one thing that I want to emphasize very strongly it is that there are no final thoughts about infertility. Reproductive medicine is making gains at an incredible rate. In writing this book I have revised it several times just on the basis of progress made during the last several months. There is no question in my mind that in the very near future, couples who are now considered very difficult to treat will be able to have babies. The future can only hold good news and more hope of a child for almost every couple who desires one. Do not give up your efforts in any way.

While you go through the diagnostic procedures to discover the reason for your infertility, it is very important that you share your feelings with your physician and with each other. The inability to produce a child when you desire it strains the very fibers of your relationship.

In past times of stress, each of you has been able to turn to your partner for emotional support. When fertility problems arise, however, you may begin to question each other's role in the predicament. Instead of being members of a couple you may become adversaries. There is a tendency for individual members of an infertile couple not to discuss their emotions. The result is an increasing feeling of isolation, frustration, hostility, and depression. To help overcome this, make your physician a partner—someone to confide in and share your problems with. Convert a tendency toward isolation into constant dialogue and sharing of feelings.

Infertility is a symptom of a medical problem. If you had a different medical problem—such as a broken arm or an ulcer—you would not be reluctant to express your feelings about it. Similarly, ideally, there should be no difference in the feelings of an infertile couple. However, because the problem involves one's own sexuality, self-value, and ego, the response is quite different. It takes a conscious effort for a man and a woman to share their feelings on this emotionally charged subject with each other and with a third person. Yet if you do, the benefits are enormous. Pressure and stress become diffused and though the problem itself may not be cured immediately, tolerating it becomes much easier.

Fifteen percent of couples of reproductive age living in the United States are unable to bear children. This means that in any group of twenty couples there is bound to be at least one, and probably three, who are infertile. Though you may feel isolated at times, you are certainly not alone. In reaching out, you will find that there are many, many people who are willing and able to help you. Besides offering medical assistance, there are also groups offering counseling and general support. Just entering a room and finding all of the individuals there sharing your problems and frustrations can change your whole outlook. It can be a totally revealing and very positive experience. RESOLVE is one such organization. (For further information, consult the appendix.)

Once a diagnosis is made you have to sit back and await the results of treatment. After many years of trying to achieve pregnancy, further waiting becomes exceedingly difficult. Nevertheless, just as the year's period of time was necessary to attempt pregnancy before treatment, very often at least this much time must be allowed to see whether or not treatment will achieve success.

One of the most difficult things to do is to wait. It is especially difficult when other couples around you are having children, most frequently without much difficulty or thought. The feelings are best handled by joining groups to share in problems and by discussing your feelings openly with your physician. In a certain sense, you have to be able to sit back and allow pregnancy to happen. I am not suggesting that you take the old "vacation cure" but I am attempting to point out that if somehow, after all of these years of effort, while therapy is started, you could maintain a dispassionate, nonjudgmental attitude, you may tolerate the time better. During this time you need to have "a place to put your head." There are various ways to diffuse some of the tension and the anxiety of this period. Counseling, consciousness-raising sessions, talking to friends and relatives, sharing your feelings, psychotherapy, and even Zen exercises, meditation, and strenuous exercise all have their roles. Each individual has to find what works for him or her.

Even if it is not possible for a couple to produce a pregnancy, it is still possible for them to have a child. Adoption can give you a child of your own as completely as by almost any other means. Love, environment, guidance, shared experiences and the fulfillment of mutual needs, all contribute to the relationship between child and parent. It becomes immaterial if the child is yours genetically or by adoption. Most areas have licensed child-placing agencies which can be helpful in arranging an adoption. In the event that this becomes too difficult because of an excessively long waiting list, occasionally an independent or private adoption through a lawyer or a physician can be arranged. Your local social service agencies and adoption bureaus can be helpful in providing information for your locality and state.

Let me say a word or two about some of the less obvious needs that drive a couple to attempt a pregnancy. Some couples desire pregnancy to hold together a failing marriage. Others consider childbearing the ultimate ego trip in that they see or hope to see little pieces of themselves carried on for future generations to admire. It is presumptuous to say that these reasons are insufficient or inappropriate for the treatment of infertility. If such couples were able to have children without medical intervention, no one would be called upon to question their needs and desires.

Most couples desire a child to make their lives more complete and to give of themselves to another individual who is uniquely theirs. But within this group there are also those who desire a pregnancy but not necessarily a child. These are highly motivated individuals who are used to attaining all goals that they have strived for and are used to overcoming barriers by sheer will and determination. Here they have reached a problem—the inability to conceive—and their natural reaction is to rise to the challenge. The need is not so much a child, but simply to succeed and produce a conception. It is very difficult to separate the couples who desire pregnancy from the couples who desire a child. Indeed, it may be the case that until pregnancy actually occurs, those who desire a pregnancy for the sake of that alone may not be aware of their feelings. The result is that at times, once pregnancy occurs, instead of feeling elation and joy, these individuals may suddenly find themselves depressed.

The issue becomes more clouded because even couples desiring a child may experience depression and some confusion of emotions with achieving a pregnancy. This is because they suddenly realize that there will be changes in their life-style, their daily lives, and their means of relating to one another for a very long time. Pregnancy and raising a family represents a very significant change from the status quo.

The point of my discussion is to emphasize that the needs of the individual couple must be constantly reevaluated throughout the entire diagnostic and treatment period. There is a point when a couple may suddenly find that their original reasons for requesting treatment no longer seem valid, but they may be somewhat ashamed or reluctant to tell their physician. You must understand that it is all right to change your mind at any time. Furthermore, it is important to realize that there are times when the evaluation and treatment of infertility may be so taxing upon both of you that the process may become worse than the problem. The "cure" becomes worse than the "disease" when evaluation and treatment begin to invade and negatively affect your private life. At that point it may be appropriate to reevaluate the situation. You may consider just "walking away" from treatment and coming back when and if things feel better. The relationship with your physician must be so close and so sensitive that, paradoxically, you must feel no qualms about stopping treatment at any time. The result is that each visit should be the product of a positive decision. It should not be carried on by rote or the inertia of a workup or treatment plan that has begun. The positive decision must be based on thorough understanding of everything that has been done and everything that will be done. It must be based on the communication between the two of you and your doctor. If you elect to stop treatment, do not make a decision at that time as to when you will return. If it feels good not to go back, that's fine. If you have a need to return, then that need will express itself in time.

Take things as they come, one thing at a time. Remember, the most complex of knots can be unraveled one step at a time by concentrating and understanding each twist and turn. If each step is understood, slow progress can be tolerated and appreciated and, in its own way, even enjoyed. Each minute in time has its own intrinsic beauty and value. It would be unfortunate to overlook it because of an unsatisfying quest. On the other hand, the future holds the answer to most of today's unanswered questions. The secret is to balance an appreciation of the present with an anticipation of the future.

Glossary

Abortion The loss of pregnancy before the fetus can survive on its own.

1. Spontaneous abortion—The loss of a pregnancy without any manipulation or administration of medication. Also called a miscarriage.

2. Induced abortion—The purposeful termination of a pregnancy by the use of instruments or medication.

3. Habitual abortion—The repetitive, consecutive, spontaneous loss of pregnancies. Evaluation for this problem used to be started after three consecutive spontaneous abortions, now the evaluation is begun after two.

4. Therapeutic abortion—An induced abortion done for medical reasons.

5. Inevitable abortion—A miscarriage diagnosed at a time when it is known that it cannot be halted.

6. Complete abortion—A miscarriage in which all of the pregnancy tissue has been expelled from the uterus. In this case a dilation and curettage is usually not needed.

7. Incomplete abortion—A miscarriage in which some of the tissue has been spontaneously expelled while some of the tissue remains in the uterus. In this case a dilation and curettage is usually needed.

8. Missed abortion—A miscarriage in which the pregnancy dies

but the tissue is not spontaneously expelled from the uterus, after four or more weeks. A dilation and curettage is usually performed to remove this tissue from the uterus.

9. Selective abortion—See "Selective Reduction."

10. Threatened abortion—A situation in early pregnancy during which the woman experiences symptoms such as vaginal bleeding with or without pain, which may end with a miscarriage or with the continuation of a normal pregnancy.

Abcess An accumulation of pus.

Adhesion Scar tissue bands attached to organ surfaces capable of connecting, covering, or distorting organs, such as Fallopian tubes, ovaries, and bowel.

Adrenal Glands Two small glands, one on the top of each kidney, which produce many of the important steroid hormones including cortisone and a normally small amount of sex hormones.

Adrenogenital Syndrome A disorder caused by a shift in the hormone production of the adrenal gland, frequently resulting in a higher production of male hormones and male secondary sex characteristics in a woman.

Agglutination of Sperm A sticking together of sperm cells.

Amenorrhea The total absence or cessation of menstrual periods for six months or more.

1. Primary Amenorrhea—The total absence of menses. A woman with primary amenorrhea has never menstruated spontaneously.

2. Secondary Amenorrhea—The total absence or cessation of menstrual periods for six months or more in a woman who previously menstruated spontaneously.

Amniocentesis Removal of a small sample of amniotic fluid from a pregnant uterus to evaluate the condition of the fetus.

Amniotic Fluid The fluid that surrounds the developing fetus in the uterus.

Ampulla In the male, a pocket of the upper end of the vas deferens in which some sperm are stored. In the female, the outer third of the Fallopian tube, which is also the portion of the tube that normally has the largest diameter.

Anastomosis A surgical procedure rejoining two separated tubal structures such as Fallopian tubes, vas deferens, or blood vessels. This procedure is usually done under microscopic magnification and thus referred to as a microsurgical anastomosis.

Androgens The general class of male sex hormones. Testosterone is the notable example.

Andrologist A physician who specializes in male reproductive problems.

Antibody A substance made by the body that normally attacks invading foreign organisms, thus preventing infection. Antibodies are directed not only at foreign substances but may be directed against parts of the human body. When antibodies destroy sperm cells, infertility may result.

Antigen Any foreign substance, frequently a microorganism, that causes the body to produce antibodies against it.

Anorexia Nervosa A potentially life-threatening eating disorder associated with a loss of appetite and excessive and dangerous weight loss. When a woman's weight falls below a certain level, ovulation problems—including luteal phase defects and total anovulation—may occur.

Anovulation The total absence of ovulation. This is not necessarily the same as "amenorrhea": menses may still occur with anovulation.

Anovulatory Bleeding Menses that occur without ovulation. The menstrual pattern is totally random, occurring at unpredictable intervals and in irregular amounts varying from spotting to major vaginal bleeding.

Artificial Insemination (AI) The introduction of sperm into a woman's vagina or cervix using an instrument rather than a penis.

1. Artificial Insemination-Homologous or Husband (AIH)—The introduction of a man's sperm into his partner's vagina or cervix using instruments in order to produce a pregnancy.

2. Artificial Insemination-Donor (AID)—The introduction of sperm from an unidentified donor into a woman's vagina or cervix using instruments, in order to produce a pregnancy.

3. Split Ejaculate Insemination—Using the first portion of the semen produced by the man for artificial insemination.

4. Intrauterine Insemination (IUI)—The introduction of sperm directly into the uterus.

Asherman's Syndrome A condition in which the walls of the uterine cavity are partially or completely stuck together by scar tissue, resulting in the partial or complete obliteration of the uterine cavity.

Asthenospermia Low sperm motility.

Azospermia The absence of sperm cells in the semen specimen.

Basal Body Temperature The body temperature of a person recorded immediately upon awakening, before activity of any kind. The temperature can be taken either orally or rectally and are recorded on a graph. The shape of the curve produced can provide some evidence of ovulation in a woman.

Benign Nonmalignant or noncancerous, usually referring to masses or tumors.

Beta HCG Test A blood or urine test used to detect the amount of Beta HCG in the blood and thus to detect very early pregnancies, and evaluate the progress of fetal development.

Bicornuate Uterus A congenital malformation of the uterus in which it is composed of two smaller horn-shaped bodies each having one Fallopian tube. This is different from a septate uterus.

Biopsy The surgical sampling or removal of tissue for examination.

Blighted Egg A general, nonspecific term used to mean a fertilized egg that fails to survive after implanting in the uterus.

Bromocryptine An oral medication used to lower prolactin levels. It can also be used to reduce the size of a pituitary tumor. This drug is sold in the United States under the name Parlodel.

Candida A yeastlike organism that can grow in the vagina—frequently producing a cottage cheese–like discharge—and is often associated with vaginal itching. Also called *monilia* or *moniliasis*.

Cannula A long, thin, hollow tube, usually attached to a syringe, used to introduce material into the body or remove material from the body.

Capacitation A change that sperm cells undergo as they travel through the woman's reproductive tract that enables the sperm to penetrate an egg.

Cauterize   To destroy tissue using heat.

Cervical Mucus   A secretion produced by the tissue lining of the cervical canal. This fluid is usually present in a small volume, but around the time of ovulation the quality of the cervical mucus changes to a large volume of watery liquid. At this time cervical mucus acts as a pathway allowing sperm cells to enter the uterus and approach an egg waiting in the Fallopian tube.

Cervical Os   The opening of the cervix. This opening connects with the cervical canal and the uterine cavity.

Cervicitis   An inflammation of the cervix. This may temporarily affect fertility.

Cervix   The lowermost portion of the uterus joining it with the vagina. A canal runs through the cervix and is continuous with the cavity of the uterus.

Cesarean Section   The delivery of a child through an incision in the uterus and the abdominal wall rather than through the vagina.

Chlamydia   A microorganism that may be transmitted by sexual contact and can be found in the genitourinary tract of men and women. Other organ systems may also be infected. In the reproductive tract, chlamydia may produce infertility.

Chocolate Cyst   A cyst in the ovary that is filled with endometriosis and has a chocolatelike, pasty appearance. Also called an endometrioma.

Chromosome   The structure in the cell that carries the genetic material. The normal human has forty-six chromosomes, twenty-three coming from the egg and twenty-three from the sperm.

Cilia   Microscopic hairlike projections from the surface of a cell capable of beating in a coordinated fashion.

Clitoris   The small erectile sex organ of the female above the urethra which contains a large numbers of sensory nerves.

Clomid   See "Clomiphene Citrate."

Clomiphene Citrate   A synthetic drug used to stimulate the hypothalamus and pituitary gland to increase FSH and LH production. It is usually used to treat anovulation but has other uses. This is the generic name for Serophene and Clomid.

Coitus Intercourse, making love, having sexual relations.

Colposcopy An examination of the cervix through a special microscope called a colposcope. This procedure frequently is used to study a cervix with an abnormal pap smear.

Conception A fetus or embryo. Sometimes called a conceptus.

Congenital A nonhereditary characteristic or defect existing since birth.

Contraception Birth control; using artificial means to prevent pregnancy.

Corpus Luteum A specialized yellow structure that forms on the surface of the ovary at the site of ovulation. It produces the progesterone characteristic of the second half of the menstrual cycle and is necessary to prepare the uterine lining for implantation by the fertilized egg.

Cortisol An important hormone produced by the adrenal glands.

Cryopreservation Preservatiuon of living tissue or cells by freezing.

Cryptorchidism The condition of having testes that have not descended from the abdomen into the scrotum.

Culdoscopy See Endoscopy.

Cushing's Disease A rare condition like Cushing's syndrome, characterized by an overproduction of adrenal hormones. Unlike the syndrome, Cushing's disease is caused by a pituitary tumor.

Cushing's Syndrome A condition characterized by an overproduction of hormones from the adrenal gland. This may be associated with decreased sperm production in men and irregular ovulation, obesity, and/or masculinization in women.

D&C See dilation and curettage.

Danazol A medication used to treat endometriosis. It suppresses LH and FSH production resulting in a decrease in ovarian estrogen production. Danazol is marketed under the names of Danocrine and Danol.

Dexamethasone A cortisonlike drug used to reduce adrenal secretions.

DHEAS A male hormone produced by the adrenal gland.

Diethylstilbestrol (DES) A synthetic estrogen prescribed in the 1950s and 1960s to women to prevent miscarriage. Some of the offspring of these pregnancies have had reproductive problems. DES is no longer prescribed for this use.

Dilation and Curettage A procedure in which the opening of the uterus, the cervix, is stretched (dilation) and the lining of the uterus scraped (curettage). Sometimes referred to as a D&C.

DNA Deoxyribonucleic acid. It is the chemical compound found within the nucleus of each cell that contains and transmits genetic information.

Down's Syndrome A birth defect usually caused by an extra chromosome in pair number 21. This genetic defect is usually associated with varying degrees of mental retardation. Also called mongolism or trisomy 21.

Doxycycline An antibiotic which is a tetracycline derivative.

Dysmenorrhea Painful menstruation.

Dyspareunia Pain on intercourse.

Ectopic Pregnancy A pregnancy that grows on a surface other than the cavity of the uterus. In most cases this condition requires surgery to remove the conceptus.
1. Tubal Pregnancy—A pregnancy in which the embryo implants in a Fallopian tube.
2. Ovarian Pregnancy—A pregnancy in which the embryo implants on the ovary.
3. Abdominal Pregnancy—A pregnancy in which the embryo implants on the surface of one of the organs in the abdomen other than the tubes or ovaries.

Egg Retrieval A procedure used to obtain eggs from ovarian follicles for use in in vitro fertilization. Egg retrieval can be done by ultrasound or laparoscopic guidance.

Ejaculation The release of seminal fluid and sperm from the penis during orgasm.

Embryo An early stage in the development of a fertilized egg, up to the eighth week of pregnancy.

Embryo Transfer A procedure used to place or insert an embryo into a woman's uterus. The embryo may be a product of in vitro fertilization, or ovum transfer.

Endocrine System   A system of ductless glands producing hormones. The system includes the pituitary, parathyroid, thyroid, and adrenal glands, the testes, and the ovaries.

Endocrinologist   A physician who specializes in the diagnosis and treatment of diseases of the hormone systems.

Endometrial Biopsy   The removal of a small sample of the lining of the uterus for microscopic examination.

Endometrioma   See "Chocolate Cyst."

Endometriosis   A condition where endometrium, the tissue which is normally found lining the uterine cavity, is found on other surfaces outside the uterus. These other surfaces may include the Fallopian tubes, ovaries, the outside surface of the uterus, and the surface of the abdominal cavity.

Endometrium   The specialized tissue layer lining the cavity of the uterus.

Endosalpinx   The specialized tissue lining the Fallopian tube.

Endoscopy   The direct viewing of the inside of the human body by the insertion of a telescopelike device into that part of the body.

1. Culdoscopy—A minor surgical procedure in which a telescopelike device is inserted through a small incision in the back of the vagina in order to look at the ovaries, Fallopian tubes, and uterus.

2. Laparoscopy—A minor surgical procedure in which a telescopelike device is inserted through a small incision in the umbilicus (the navel) in order to view the abdominal contents including the ovaries, Fallopian tubes, and uterus. Limited surgery may also be done with this procedure.

3. Hysteroscopy—A minor surgical procedure in which a telescopelike device is inserted through the cervix into the cavity of the uterus in order to directly view the entire cavity. Limited surgery may also be done with this procedure. An incision is not needed to insert the telescope.

Epididymis   A coiled tubular structure in the male which receives sperm from the testes. The sperm is stored, nourished, and matured for a period of several months, then conducted into the vas deferens.

Epispadius A congenital abnormality of the penis, in which the opening of the urethra is on the top of the penis instead of at the end.

Erection The state where the penis, when aroused, is engorged, erect, and somewhat rigid.

Estrogen The primary female hormone. It is a steroid hormone produced mainly by the ovaries from puberty to menopause and in lesser amounts by the adrenal gland and fatty tissue.

Fallopian Tubes Paired hollow tubular structures found extending from the body of the uterus toward the ovaries. These structures pick up the egg through their funnel-shaped ends and conduct it to the uterus. Fertilization takes place within this structure. Also called the oviduct.

Fertility The ability of a heterosexual couple to produce offspring.

Fertility Specialist A physician specializing in the practice of fertility. Within this category there is a group of physicians who have been specially trained in reproductive medicine and certified after extensive testing by the American Board of Obstetrics and Gynecology. These are certified subspecialists in reproductive endocrinology and infertility. A list of these physicians is available from the American College of Obstetrics and Gynecology. These subspecialists are not the only doctors capable of adequately treating infertile couples.

Fertilization The union of a sperm and an egg by penetration.

Fetal Loss A term often used to include both miscarriage and stillbirth.

Fetus The stage of development of an animal or human pregnancy while still in the uterus from the third month until delivery.

Fibroid Tumor A benign (noncancerous) tumor found within the wall of the uterus, sometimes distorting uterine and/or tubal anatomy. Also known as a myoma.

Fimbria The fluted, funnel-shaped outermost portion of the Fallopian tube, specialized in egg pickup.

Follicle   The structure in the ovary that nurtures the ripening egg and from which the egg is released.

Follicle-Stimulating Hormone (FSH)   A hormone produced and released from the pituitary gland. In the female it stimulates estrogen production and development of follicles in the ovary. Follicular stimulation by FSH is necessary to prepare for ovulation. In the male, FSH stimulates sperm production.

Follicular Phase   The first portion of the menstrual cycle occurring from the beginning of the menstrual cycle to just prior to ovulation during which time the follicle develops and the egg matures.

Frigidity   The inability of a woman to experience sexual arousal.

FSH   An abbreviation for follicle-stimulating hormone. See "Follicle-Stimulating Hormone."

Galactorrhea   A milky discharge from the breasts which may be associated with an elevated prolactin level and infertility.

Gamete   A sperm or an egg.

Gamete Intra-Fallopian Tube Transfer (GIFT)   A procedure usually done to treat infertility in couples with infertility of undetermined origin. The woman is given ovulation-stimulation medication in a manner similar to that for in vitro fertilization. A laparoscopy is performed, eggs retrieved and mixed with a suspension of sperm, the mixture loaded into a long plastic tube, and—during the same laparoscopy—injected back into the woman's Fallopian tube. This can be done only in women with normal Fallopian tubes.

Genes   Structures within the nucleus of each cell that convey hereditary characteristics, consisting primarily of DNA and proteins and occurring at specific points on the chromosomes.

Genetic   Referring to characteristics transmitted by heredity.

Genetic Abnormality   A disorder arising from an abnormality or error in the chromosomal or gene structure which may be hereditary.

Genetic Counseling   Advice and information provided, usually by a team of specialists, on the detection and risk of recurrence of genetic disorders and fetal abnormalities.

Genetic Studies   Laboratory studies allowing the identification of certain abnormal states and hereditary disorders. This is usually done by studying certain tissues or white blood cells. The tests are also known as karyotyping.

Gestation The period of fetal development in the uterus from conception to birth. This is usually forty weeks in human pregnancies.

Gland A hormone-producing organ.

Gonads A general term referring to the glands which make reproductive cells. The testes in the male and ovaries in the female.

Gonadotropin-Releasing Hormone(GnRH) A substance produced by the hypothalamus in bursts approximately every ninety minutes which enables the pituitary to secrete LH and FSH in the appropriate way. Also called luteinizing hormone-releasing hormone, or factor. This hormone is abbreviated as GnRH, LHRH, and LRF.

Gonadotropins Pituitary hormones FSH and LH, which biochemically stimulate the testes or ovaries.

Gonorrhea A highly contagious disease caused by gonococcus bacteria which affects the male and female reproductive systems. Other organ systems may be involved. The disease is spread mainly through sexual intercourse and can affect fertility.

Gynecologist A physician who specializes in the diagnosis and treatment of diseases of the female reproductive system.

HCG An abbreviation for human chorionic gonadotropin. See "Human Chorionic Gonadotropin."

Hirsutism Excessive hair growth, usually in women.

HMG An abbreviation for human menopausal gonadotropin. This fertility drug, marketed in the United States under the name of Pergonal, is FSH and LH extracted from urine of menopausal women. It is an injectable drug used to stimulate ovulation in women and is capable of stimulating sperm production in some men.

Hormone A chemical produced by a ductless gland of the body.

Hostility Factor A condition that results in the lack of survival of sperm cells in vaginal or cervical fluids. It manifests itself as a poor postcoital test.

Huhner Test See "Postcoital Test."

Human Chorionic Gonadotropin (HCG)   A hormone produced by the human placenta which maintains the corpus luteum beyond its usual fourteen-day life span. The result is a continual source of progesterone to support an early pregnancy. This hormone may be injected following HMG to trigger ovulation. It is also the basis of most pregnancy tests.

Human Menopausal Gonadotropin (HMG)   The generic name for Pergonal. This is an extract of menopausal urine containing FSH and LH. HMG is administered by injection to treat certain types of anovulation in women and azospermia or oligospermia in men.

Husband Artificial Insemination   See "Artificial Insemination."

Hydrosalpinx   A large, fluid filled, club-shaped Fallopian tube closed at the fimbriated end (at the end closest to the ovary). It is a cause of infertility.

Hydrotubation   A procedure whereby the Fallopian tubes are flushed with a sterile solution injected through the cervix. The solution may or may not have medication in it. Its role in the treatment of infertility is controversial. Also known as hydropertubation, pertubation, and tubal lavage.

Hymen   A membranous covering at the opening of the vagina. Its thickness may vary from woman to woman. If it is thin enough it will break with first complete vaginal penetration. If it is quite thick, surgical removal may be necessary.

Hyperstimulation   A condition that exists when a large number of follicles are stimulated to develop and ovulate, resulting in an enlargement of the ovaries. When this enlargement is massive, hospitalization is necessary. Hyperstimulation is a potential risk of Pergonal use. The risks of developing this condition can be minimized with careful monitoring.

Hypospadias   A malformation of the penis in which the urethral opening, through which urine and sperm leave the penis, is found on the underside rather than the tip of the penis.

Hypothalamus   The region of the brain just above the pituitary that controls hormone production and release by the pituitary gland.

Hypothyroidism   A state of reduced thyroid function.

Hysterectomy   The surgical removal of the uterus.

Hysterosalpingogram   An X-ray procedure that is done by injecting a dye which can be seen on X-ray through the cervix into the uterus and tubes. It is frequently performed to see if the Fallopian tubes are open and if the uterine cavity is of normal shape. Also called a uterotubogram, or hysterogram, and abbreviated as HSG.

Hysteroscopy   See "Endoscopy."

Hysterotomy   A surgical procedure in which an incision is made in the uterus and is later closed after appropriate uterine reconstruction or repair is performed.

Implantation   The adhering of a fertilized egg to the lining of the uterus.

Impotence   The inability of a male to have or maintain an erection of his penis.

Incompetent Cervix   A condition in which the cervix of a pregnant uterus opens prematurely, allowing the fetus to slip out. This usually occurs during the second or third trimester and can be a cause of pregnancy loss or premature delivery.

Infertility   The inability of a heterosexual couple to conceive after one year of regular unprotected intercourse.

1. Primary Infertility—The inability of a couple to conceive after one year of regular unprotected intercourse, with no previous pregnancies having occurred.

2. Secondary Infertility—Infertility occurring after at least one successful pregnancy and delivery.

Insufflation of the Tubes   See "Rubin Test."

Interstitial Cell   See "Leydig Cells."

Intrauterine   Inside the uterus.

In Vitro Fertilization   A procedure in which an egg is removed from a ripe follicle and fertilized by a sperm cell outside the human body. The fertilized egg is allowed to divide in a protected environment for about two days and then is transferred into the uterus of the woman who produced the egg. Also called "test-tube fertilization."

Karyotype   See "Genetic Studies."

Klinefelter's Syndrome   A condition in which a male has XXY sex chromosomes instead of XY. A man with this condition is usually sterile.

Laparoscopy See "Endoscopy."

Laparotomy Abdominal surgery.

Leydig Cells Cells in the testes that produce testosterone. Also called interstitial cells.

LHRH Another abbreviation for GnRH. See "Gonadotropin-Releasing Hormone."

LH Surge A sudden, massive release of LH from the pituitary gland at midcycle resulting in the release of an egg from the ovary (ovulation).

Libido Sexual desire.

Luteal Phase The last fourteen days of an ovulatory cycle, associated with progesterone production.

Luteal Phase Defect A condition in which the lining of the uterus does not develop properly because of a partial deficiency of progesterone. This may result in infertility or early pregnancy loss. Abbreviated as LPD.

Luteinized Unruptured Follicle Syndrome A condition in which all of the clinical signs that indicate ovulation are present (blood hormonal changes, temperature rise on basal body temperature chart, as well as endometrial biopsy changes), but the egg is never actually released from the surface of the ovary. The egg remains trapped in the follicle. This syndrome is treatable with clomiphene or Pergonal. Abbreviated as LUF.

Luteinizing Hormone A hormone produced and released by the pituitary gland. In the female it is responsible for ovulation and the maintenance of the corpus luteum for progesterone production. In the male it stimulates testosterone production and is important in spermatogenesis (the production of sperm cells). Abbreviated as LH.

Lysis of Adhesions A surgical procedure in which scar tissue on the surface of organs is removed.

Menarche The age at which a female has her first menstrual flow (period).

Menopause The time of a woman's last "regular" menstrual flow, which marks the beginning of the failure of the ovary.
   1. Physiologic Menopause—Menopause occurring spontaneously. The normal cessation of ovarian function, usually be-

tween age forty-five and fifty. Also known as the "change of life."

2. Surgical Menopause—Menopause resulting from the surgical removal of the ovaries.

Menorrhagia Heavy menstrual bleeding.

Menses A woman's period or menstrual flow.

Menstruation The regular shedding of the lining of the uterus, usually resulting in cyclic monthly vaginal bleeding. This process occurs in the absence of pregnancy from menarche to menopause.

Metrorrhagia Prolonged menstrual bleeding or bleeding between menstrual periods.

Microsurgery Reconstructive surgery done with the aid of magnification, frequently with a microscope, using extremely fine suture material with very gentle manipulation of the tissue. The result when applied to Fallopian tube or vas deferens surgery appears to be a significant increase in successful reconstruction.

Miscarriage See "Abortion."

Mittelschmertz Pain felt by some women at midcycle during ovulation. It is not absolute proof of ovulation nor is its absence proof that ovulation does not occur.

Morphology of Sperm The study of the shape of sperm cells. This evaluation is part of a semen analysis.

Motility of Sperm The ability of sperm cells to move. This evaluation is part of a sperm analysis.

Mutagen A substance that alters the genetic structure of a cell.

Mycoplasma See "Ureaplasma."

Myoma A common benign tumor of the muscle of the uterus. This is sometimes called a fibroid. See "Fibroid Tumor."

Myomectomy The surgical removal of fibroid tumors from the wall of the uterus.

Nidation See "Implantation."

Obstetrician A physician who treats pregnant women, provides care for the fetus, and manages labor and the delivery of the baby.

Oligomenorrhea Infrequent menstrual periods.

Oligospermia A scarcity of sperm in a semen sample.

Oocyte An egg or an ovum.

Oral Contraceptive A drug taken by mouth to prevent pregnancy by suppressing ovulation.

Orchitis An inflammation of the testes.

Orgasm The moment of highest sexual excitement. In the male this is marked by ejaculation. In the female this is a time of pleasure with a series of muscular contractions of the pelvic muscles.

Ovarian Dysgenesis See "Turner's Syndrome."

Ovarian Failure A condition that exists when the ovary has no more follicles and thus does not respond to FSH stimulation from the pituitary gland. This is usually associated with an elevation of FSH and LH levels.

Ovary The female sex gland with both a reproductive function (releasing eggs) and a hormonal function (producing estrogen and progesterone).

Oviduct See "Fallopian Tube."

Ovulation The release of a mature egg from the surface of the ovary.

Ovulation Induction Medical treatment to produce ovulation.

Ovum An egg.

Ovum Transfer Process by which artificial insemination of a woman results in an embryo that is flushed out of the uterus of one woman after conception and implanted in a second woman, the partner of the man who donated the sperm.

Pap Test A screening test to examine a woman for the presence of cervical cancer. It is done by gently touching a cotton swab on the cervix and then wiping the swab on a slide which is treated and examined under a microscope.

Patent The condition of being open, as with tubes that form part of the reproductive organs. Fallopian tubes that allow dye to pass through them, demonstrating that they are not closed, are said to be "patent."

Pelvic Inflammatory Disease (PID) A generalized infection of the pelvis or female reproductive organs.

Penis The male organ used for sexual intercourse and urination.

Pergonal   The brand name under which human menopausal gonadotropin (HMG) is sold.

Perinatal   Referring to the period of time from the twentieth week of pregnancy through the first twenty-eight days of life.

Peritoneal Cavity   The abdominal cavity.

Peritoneum   The lining of the abdominal cavity.

Peritubal Adhesions   Connective tissue bands around the Fallopian tubes, sometimes immobilizing or obstructing the tubes. The result may be a disturbance in egg pickup and infertility.

Pituitary Gland   A gland located at the base of the brain, below the hypothalamus, which controls almost every endocrine gland in the body. Also known as the "master gland," it controls human growth, development, functioning, and reproduction.

Pneumoperitoneum   The introduction of gas into the peritoneal cavity. This is usually done with laparoscopy.

Polycystic Ovary Syndrome   A condition in which a woman has enlarged ovaries containing multiple cysts and a thickened coat on the surface of the ovary. The woman usually ovulates infrequently or not at all. Stein-Leventhal syndrome is a form of Polycystic ovary syndrome.

Postcoital   Referring to after intercourse.

Postcoital Test   The microscopic study of samples of vaginal and cervical secretions taken several hours after sexual relations. The physician looks for moving, apparently live, sperm cells. Also known as the Sims-Huhner Test, the P.K. test, and the P.C. test.

Prednisone   A cortisonelike drug used to reduce adrenal secretions.

Premature Ejaculation   The release of sperm from the penis prior to or immediately after entering the vagina.

Premature Menopause   Ovarian failure occurring before age forty.

Progesterone   A hormone produced and released by the corpus luteum of the ovary during the second half of an ovulatory cycle. It is necessary for the preparation of the lining of the uterus for the implantation of the fertilized egg. It is also produced by the placenta during pregnancy.

Prostate Gland A gland that surrounds the male urethra at its exit from the bladder and contributes secretions to the seminal fluid.

Puberty The age at which the testes and ovaries begin to function. At this time the young man or woman develops the appropriate sexual characteristics and conception becomes possible.

Resistant Ovary An ovary that contains follicles but does not respond to the usual levels of FSH and LH stimulation. Occasionally very high levels of FSH and LH will produce ovulation.

Retrograde Ejaculation A condition in which sperm flows backward into the bladder instead of out through the penis during ejaculation.

Retroverted Uterus A uterus tilted backward toward the woman's back rather than the more common state of tilting toward the front of the abdomen. By itself this should not be a cause of infertility. Also known as a "tilted" or "tipped" uterus.

Rubin Test A test to demonstrate that the Fallopian tubes are open. Carbon dioxide, a gas, is passed into the uterus and its pressure measured. If the tubes are open, the gas will leak out and the pressure will remain low. The woman will complain of shoulder pain if the tubes are not completely obstructed.

Salpingectomy The surgical removal of the Fallopian tube.

Salpingitis An inflammation of the Fallopian tubes, usually due to infection.

Salpingogram See "Hysterosalpingogram."

Salpingolysis The surgical removal of bands of scar tissue, called adhesions, from around the Fallopian tubes. These adhesions restrict the movement of the tubes and may act as obstacles to egg pickup.

Salpingo-oophorectomy The surgical removal of a Fallopian tube and ovary, together.

Salpingoplasty See "Tuboplasty."

Salpingostomy A surgical procedure to open the Fallopian tube when it is closed at its outer end. This procedure is used to reconstruct a hydrosalpinx.

Scrotum A sac composed mainly of skin, found below the penis, which holds the testes.

Secondary Infertility See "Infertility."

Secretory Phase That portion of the menstrual cycle occurring after ovulation and prior to the onset of menses.

Selective Reduction The selective termination of one or more embryos in the face of a large number of multiple pregnancies in one woman. The remaining embryos usually continue to survive well. This procedure is performed on a woman, at her request, who has four or more embryos growing inside her uterus. This is done because of the significant risk to both the mother and babies associated with a large number of multiple births.

Semen The liquid secretions and sperm cells that are released from the penis during ejaculation.

Semen Analysis The microscopic study of a fresh semen sample. The fluid volume is measured. The number of sperm cells per unit of volume is counted and expressed as millions of cells per cubic centimeter. The percentage of normally shaped cells and percentage of moving cells are also reported.

Seminiferous Tubules Structures within the testes that produce sperm cells.

Septum An abnormality in organ structure present since birth in which a wall is present where one should not exist.
1. Septate Uterus—A uterus with a wall projecting into its cavity.
2. Vaginal Septum—A wall dividing the vagina lengthwise or obstructing it with a side-to-side placement.

Serophene See "Clomiphene Citrate."

Short Luteal Phase A variety of luteal phase defect.

Sims-Huhner Test See "Postcoital Test."

Sperm Antibodies Antibodies against sperm cells that may attack and destroy these cells. These antibodies can be produced either by men against their own sperm or by women.

Sperm Bank A registered tissue bank that, for a fee, collects, stores, tests, and disseminates sperm for artificial insemination.

Sperm Morphology The study of the shape and structure of sperm cells.

Spermatogenesis The production of sperm cells.

Spermatozoa Male reproductive cells. Also known as sperm cells.

Spinnbarkeit The stretchability of cervical mucus. This is a rough measure of how easily sperm cells can enter and penetrate the cervical secretions.

Split Ejaculate A method of collecting a semen specimen so that the first half of the ejaculate is caught in one container and the rest in a second container. In most men the first specimen will contain the vast majority of the sperm. This first portion can then be used to inseminate the woman.

Stein-Levinthal Disease See "Polycystic Ovary Syndrome."

Surrogate Mother A woman who agrees to carry and deliver a child for another woman.

Test-tube Baby A popular term for the production of a pregnancy through the fertilization of an egg outside the human body. See "In Vitro Fertilization."

Testicle See "Testis."

Testis The male sex gland with both a reproductive function (producing sperm cells) and a hormone function (producing testosterone).

Testicular Biopsy A minor surgical procedure in which a small piece of a testis is removed for microscopic study. This is usually reserved for a male who has extremely low or absent sperm production.

Testosterone A steroid hormone, made by the testes, which is the most potent male sex hormone.

Thyroid Gland A gland in the neck which produces thyroid hormone.

Thyroxin One of the hormones of the thyroid gland.

"Tipped Uterus" See "Retroverted Uterus."

Tissue Typing A procedure for testing and matching tissue and organs in a way similar to typing blood. With blood, ABO and Rh typing is used. With tissue type the HLA system is used.

T-mycoplasma One strain of ureaplasma. See "Ureaplasma."

Toxemia An abnormal condition of late pregnancy characterized by generalized swelling, high blood pressure, and protein in the urine. In an uncontrolled state it can progress to convulsions in the pregnant woman.

Toxoplasma An organism that may infect women during pregnancy, possibly causing abortion or brain damage in the fetus.

Trichomonas An organism that may be transferred during sexual intercourse. It may cause a foamy vaginal discharge, vaginal burning, and itching.

Tubal Insufflation See "Rubin Test."

Tuboplasty A general term referring to any surgical reconstruction of the Fallopian tube. Also known as salpingoplasty.

Turner's Syndrome An abnormality of genetic material in which a female has XO sex chromosomes instead of the normal XX. Most women with this condition are sterile.

Ultrasound A diagnostic technique that uses sound waves to visualize structures inside the body. The image is displayed on a video screen and can be recorded on film or videotape.

Umbilicus The navel or belly button.

Ureaplasma (Mycoplasma) A microorganism that may be associated with infertility and/or miscarriage.

Urethra The channel draining the urinary bladder. In the male it is the passage within the penis which carries, at different times, urine and semen.

Urologist A physician who diagnoses and treats diseases of the male or female urinary tract and treats problems of the male reproductive tract.

Uterus A hollow, muscular structure, part of the female reproductive tract, that is the source of a woman's menses. Its prime reproductive function is to house, protect, and nourish the developing fetus.

Vagina A tubular passageway in the female connecting the external sex organs with the cervix and uterus. Also known as the "birth canal".

Vaginismus A condition in which there is an extreme tightening of the muscles about the opening of the vagina, making the insertion of a penis during sexual relations painful, difficult, or impossible.

Varicocele   A varicose vein around the vas deferens and the testis. This may be a cause of male infertility.

Varicocelectomy   A surgical procedure that corrects a varicocele.

Vas Deferens   A thick-walled tubular structure running from each testis into the ejaculatory duct. This structure carries sperm from the epididymis to the penis.

Vasectomy   A minor surgical procedure done to interrupt and obstruct the vas deferens, a male sterilization procedure.

Vasogram   An X-ray of sperm ducts.

Venereal Disease   Any infection transmitted by sexual intercourse. VD is a major cause of infertility in both men and women if untreated, but it is readily treatable if diagnosed and treated early.

Viability   When referring to a fetus, this term refers to the capability of surviving outside the uterus. This is usually thought to be, at the earliest, twenty weeks of gestation.

Virilization   A masculinization or male type of appearance of a woman associated with an excess of male hormone.

Wedge Resection   A surgical procedure in which a wedge-shaped section of an ovary is removed and the opening created is sutured closed.

Zygote   A fertilized egg.

APPENDIX I
Numbers and Normals

I. Statistics
   A. Sixty to eighty percent of couples of reproductive age who undergo a complete infertility evaluation conceive with treatment.

   Five percent of infertile couples become pregnant without therapy.

   B. The following are pregnancy rates of sexually active women of childbearing age:

   after one month of sexual relations—25 percent will be pregnant

   after six months—63 percent will be pregnant

   after nine months—75 percent will be pregnant

   after twelve months—80 percent will be pregnant

   after eighteen months—90 percent will be pregnant

   C. Fifteen percent of couples of reproductive age in the United States are infertile. That is approximately one couple in six. The actual number is in excess of ten million people.

   D. Causes of Infertility

   40 percent—male factor

   50 percent—female factor

   15 percent anovulation

   30 percent tubal problem

   5 percent cervical problem

Ten percent—no cause can be found. (Note that in a recent study the percentage of unexplained infertility was reduced to 3.5 percent.)

E. More than 90 percent of couples who are completely evaluated can find a cause for their infertility; 50 to 60 percent will conceive.

F. Ninety-five percent of women who are anovulatory will be made to ovulate by drug treatment. About 50 percent will conceive.

II. Normal values for a semen analysis—in our laboratory count—more than 20 million cells/milliliter with a mean of 40–80 million cells/milliliter.

Volume—2–5 milliliter

Motility at two hours—more than 50 percent

Morphology—more than 60 percent normal forms

Fructose—present

Note that sperm count may vary in the same patient from ejaculate to ejaculate by 20 percent. Furthermore, even counting the same specimen several times may be associated with an error of 10 percent.

HYSTEROSALPINGOGRAM

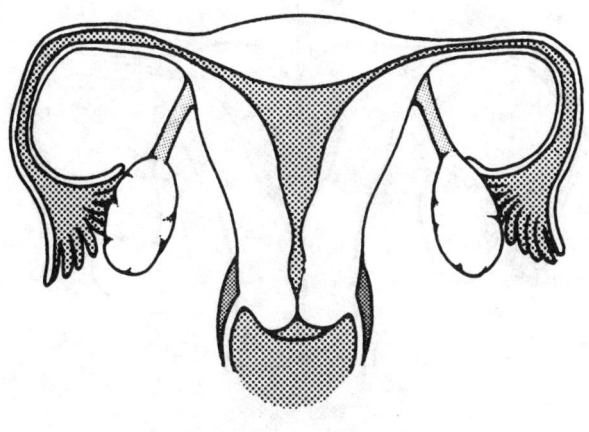

anatomy

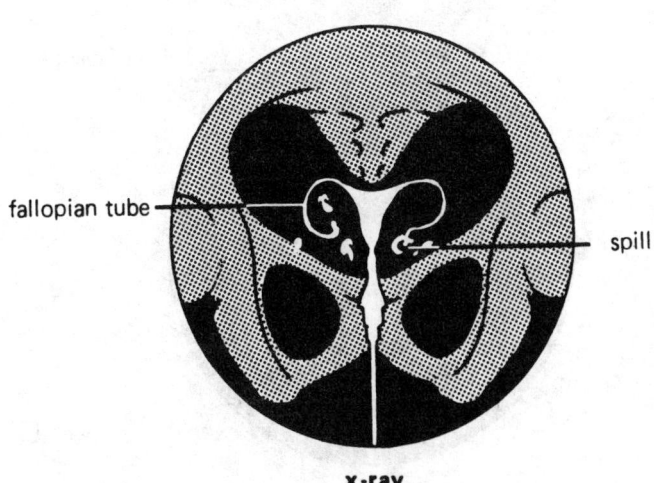

fallopian tube

spill

x-ray

NORMAL

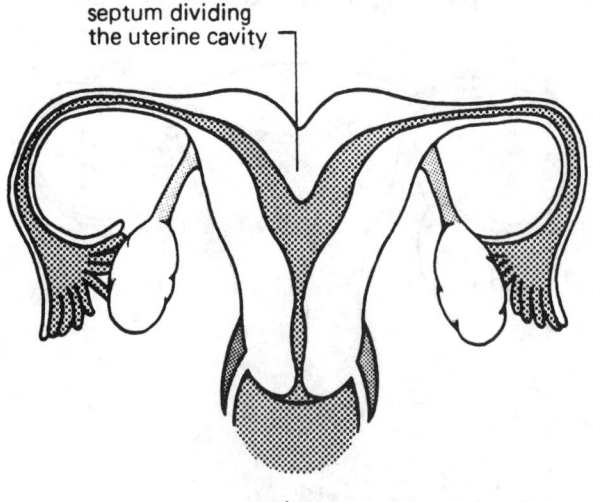

septum dividing
the uterine cavity

anatomy

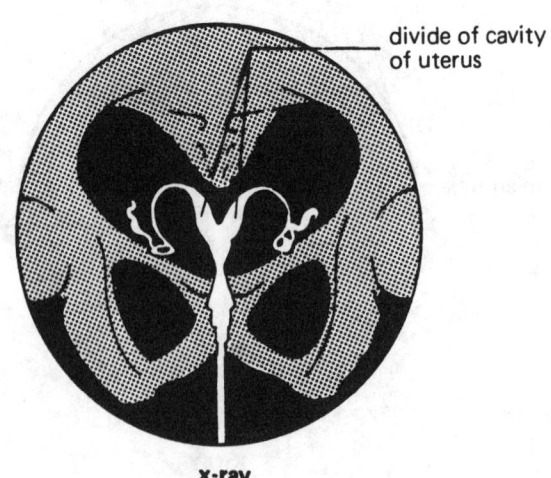

divide of cavity
of uterus

x-ray

SEPTUM

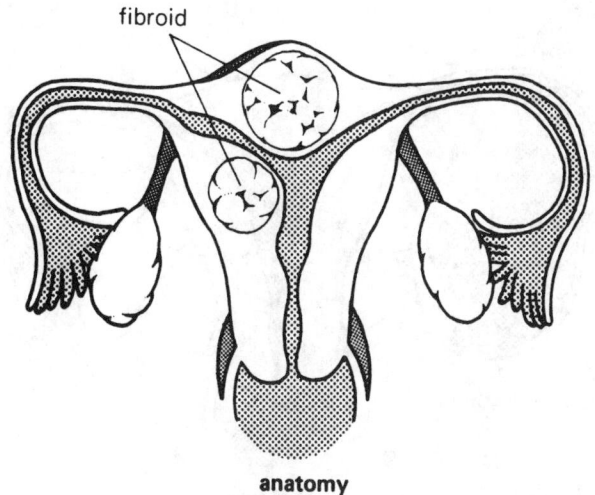

fibroid

anatomy

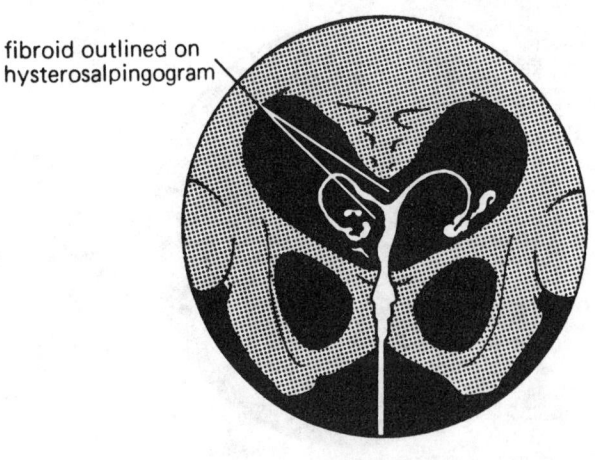

fibroid outlined on
hysterosalpingogram

x-ray

FIBROID

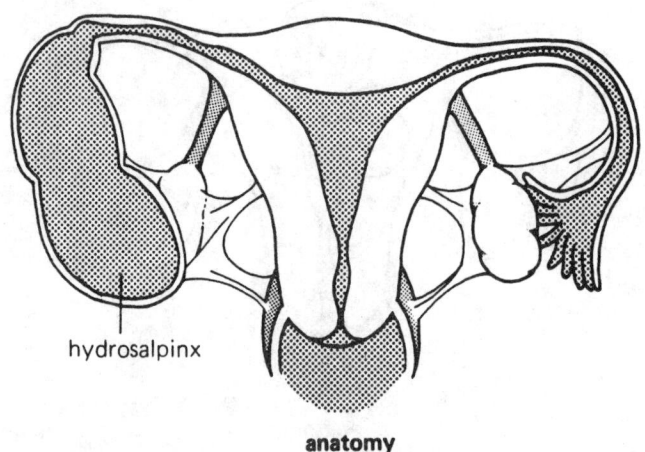

hydrosalpinx

anatomy

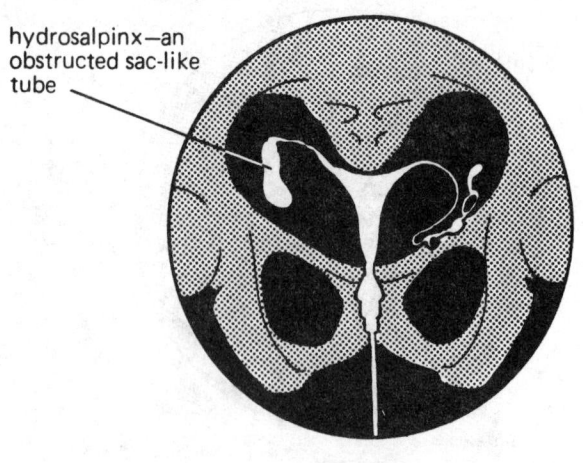

hydrosalpinx—an
obstructed sac-like
tube

x-ray

HYDROSALPINX

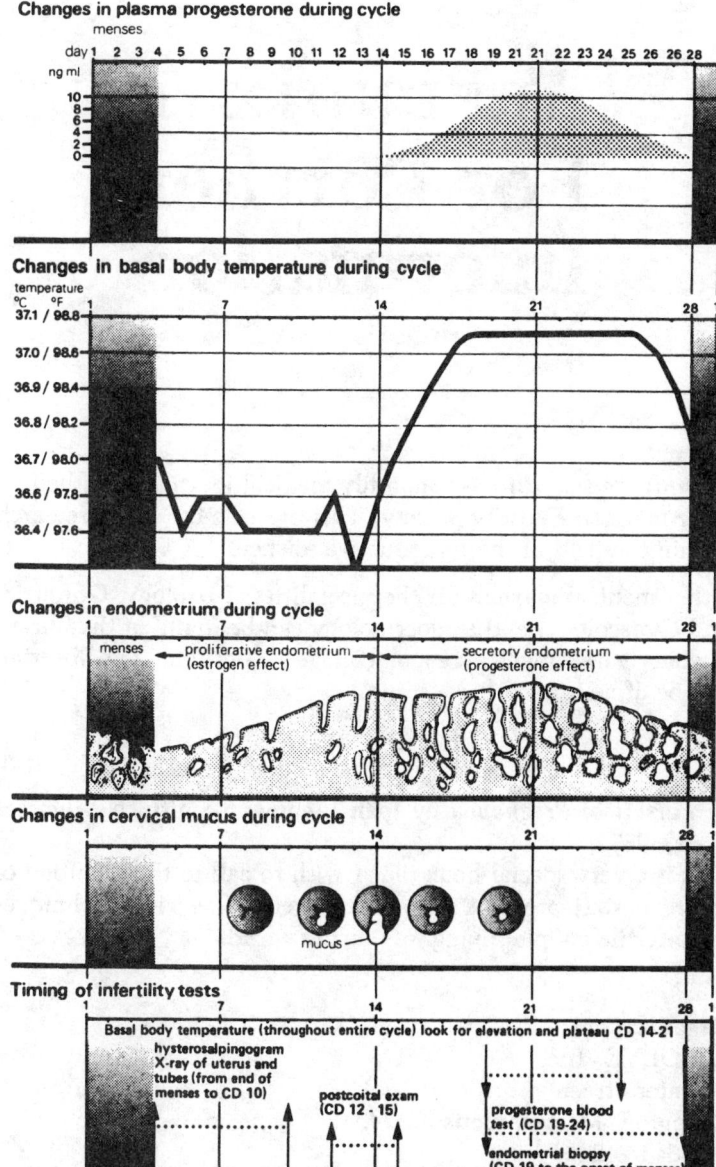

Changes in plasma progesterone during cycle

Changes in basal body temperature during cycle

Changes in endometrium during cycle

menses ← proliferative endometrium → (estrogen effect) | secretory endometrium (progesterone effect)

Changes in cervical mucus during cycle

mucus

Timing of infertility tests

Basal body temperature (throughout entire cycle) look for elevation and plateau CD 14-21

hysterosalpingogram
X-ray of uterus and tubes (from end of menses to CD 10)

postcoital exam
(CD 12 - 15)

progesterone blood test (CD 19-24)

endometrial biopsy
(CD 19 to the onset of menses)

APPENDIX II

For Further Information

Journals
Fertility and Sterility—a monthly medical journal published by the American Fertility Society. This presents the latest research within the field of the reproductive sciences.

Other medical journals for the specialities of Urology, Obstetrics and Gynecology, and Endocrinology can be found at the library of your nearest medical school, college, or hospital. The librarian can be of assistance.

Books
In Pursuit of Pregnancy by Joan Liebmann-Smith, Newmarket Press, 1987.
This is a very special book that I wish to call to the attention of the reader. It provides support and general survival techniques for infertile couples living in a fertile world.

Organizations
RESOLVE, Inc.
5 Water Street
Arlington, Massachusetts 02174
617-643-2424
A nonprofit organization directed toward the help and support

of the infertile couple. Counseling, support groups, medical information, and a local referral service are part of its work.

American Fertility Society
1608 13th Avenue, South
Suite 101
Birmingham, Alabama 35205
205-251-9764
This organization is a source of specialists from which you may choose a specialist in infertility.

American Association of Gynecologic Laparoscopists
13021 East Florence Avenue
Santa Fe Springs, California 90670
213-946-8774
This organization can act as a source of names of specialists from which you may choose a specialist in infertility.

Planned Parenthood Federation of America
810 Seventh Avenue
New York, New York 10019
212-541-7800
This organization can act as a source of information about reproductive problems in general and may be able to provide specific information about health care in various communities.

Adoption
For those for whom adoption is an appropriate choice, I hope the following information will be of assistance. Before beginning the adoption process I strongly advise that you consult the following books:

Successful Adoption: A Guide to Finding a Child and Raising a Family, by Jacqueline Hornor Plumez, Harmony Books, 1982.

The Adoption Resources Book: A Comprehensive Guide to All the Things You Need to Know and Ought to Know About Creating an Adoptive Family, by Lois Gilman, Harper & Row, 1977.

An Adoptor's Advocate, by Patricia Irwin Johnston, Perspective Press, 1984.

There are three types of adoption: domestic, international, and private. Each one has its own sources of information.

DOMESTIC ADOPTION
- Consult your local child welfare department or bureau of social services.
- Call or write:
  Adoptive Parents Committee, Inc.
  210 Fifth Avenue
  New York, New York 10010
  (212) 683-9221
- Contact your local church or temple, or contact an adoptive agency associated with your religious preferences.
  Betheny Christian Services
  (Consult your local phone book.)
  Catholic Family Services
  (Consult your local phone book.)
  Jewish Family Services
  (Consult your local phone book.)

INTERNATIONAL ADOPTION
- Contact:
  International Concerns Committee for Children (ICCC)
  Anna Marie Merrill
  911 Cypress Drive
  Boulder, Colorado 80303
  For $5.00 they will send you a booklet entitled *Report on Foreign Adoption*, which is the most comprehensive listing of active and competent foreign agencies as well as direct adoption sources.
- Write:
  Holt International Children's Service, Inc.
  P. O. Box 2886
  Eugene, Oregon 97402

PRIVATE ADOPTION
- Contact:
  Adoptive Parents Committee, Inc.
  210 Fifth Avenue

New York, New York 10010
(212) 683-9221
This organization can provide a list of attorneys who they feel are current in the knowledge of state adoption laws.

Be careful with private adoptions before "investing" your emotions and your money. Check your sources carefully.

INDEX

(Page numbers set in italics refer to illustrations.)